FAST FACTS

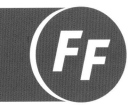

Breast Cancer *ASH*

Third edition

All You Need to Keep up to Speed

Michael Baum MD ChM FRCS FRCR FRSA
Professor Emeritus of Surgery and
Visiting Professor of Medical Humanities
University College London, London, UK

Harvey Schipper BASc(Eng) MD FRCP(C)
Professor of Medicine
University of Toronto
Toronto, Ontario, Canada

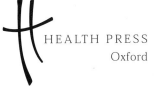

HEALTH PRESS
Oxford

Declara
This book
can make
welcome:

Fast Facts – Breast Cancer
First published 1998
Second edition August 2002
Third edition May 2005

Text © 2005 Michael Baum, Harvey Schipper
© 2005 in this edition Health Press Limited
Health Press Limited, Elizabeth House, Queen Street, Abingdon,
Oxford OX14 3LN, UK
Tel: +44 (0)1235 523233
Fax: +44 (0)1235 523238

Book orders can be placed by telephone or via the website.
For regional distributors or to order via the website, please go to: www.fastfacts.com
For telephone orders, please call 01752 202301 (UK) or
800 538 1287 (North America, toll free).

Fast Facts is a trademark of Health Press Limited.

A CIP catalogue record for this title is available from the British Library.

ISBN 1-903734-62-2

Baum M (Michael)
Fast Facts – Breast Cancer /
Michael Baum, Harvey Schipper

Medical illustrations by Dee McLean, London, UK, and
Annamaria Dutto, Withernsea, UK.
Typesetting and page layout by Zed, Oxford, UK.
Printed by Fine Print (Services) Ltd, Oxford, UK.

Printed with vegetable inks on fully biodegradable and
recyclable paper manufactured from sustainable forests.

Low emissions
during production

Low
chlorine

Sustainable
forests

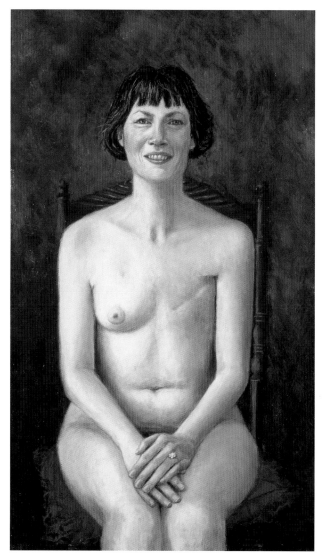

There is life after mastectomy. Portrait by Heath Rosselli, reproduced by kind permission of the artist.

Introduction

Progress in breast cancer does not come easily. The disease has a very long and unpredictable natural history. Certainly, at a biological and molecular level, we can accumulate 'facts' rapidly, but to translate these facts into valuable clinical outcomes is a very slow and painstaking process. For example, we may have a treatment that could genuinely reduce mortality from breast cancer by about 30%, but it would take a clinical trial involving several thousand women and 10 years' follow-up to detect such an important improvement.

The past few years have offered the beginnings of a fundamental change. Our conceptual understanding of malignancy is evolving from that of a pathological entity to that of a regulatory process. As a consequence, the period for intervention extends from the time preventative measures are taken, years before a clinical tumor is likely to appear, to long after local resection of an obvious mass. This has significant implications for both the patient and the healthcare system, as the net effect is to increase the number of patients and extend the period of follow-up.

The emerging consumerism in medicine is also bringing about change. Patients want to know more and to assume a less passive role in their medical management. Cancer centers are no longer just venues for treatment, but are becoming regional resources offering guidance in decision-making and providing data for evaluation. The need to balance choices is a theme repeated throughout the book, and *Fast Facts – Breast Cancer* attempts to provide a context for putting the risks and benefits into perspective. The purpose of this book is to sort out the facts from the fancies and fallacies, and to provide the busy clinician or clinical nurse specialist with rapid access to information that will make their difficult and delicate task that much easier. We owe it to our patients to provide them with comprehensive care and must make every effort to maintain their integration within the community throughout the course of a chronic illness.

Breast cancer is the most common form of cancer among women in industrialized countries, accounting for about 18% of all female cancers. Although mortality is declining in some countries, breast cancer remains the leading cause of death among women aged 35–55 years. In the UK, for example, it causes about 13 000 deaths each year, and about 35 000 new cases are diagnosed annually, while in the USA, there are about 217 500 new cases and 40 580 deaths. Sadly, even as deaths from breast cancer fall in the UK and North America, deaths from lung cancer are rising as the population of young women who embraced the tobacco habit reaches middle age, an observation all the more frustrating as lung cancer is a preventable disease.

Classical epidemiological studies repeated worldwide have established risk associations with breast cancer. These associations have been bolstered by laboratory tissue and animal studies. The following observations, which were made before the advent of contemporary molecular genetics, continue to hold true.

The incidence of breast cancer increases with age; approximately 50% of breast cancers occur in women aged 50–64 years, and a further 30% occur in women over the age of 70 years. There are also marked geographical variations in incidence; in general, the highest incidences are seen in Western countries, and the lowest in Asian and African countries (Figure 1.1). This illustrates the importance of environmental risk factors, as women from low-risk countries, such as Japan, who emigrate to higher-risk countries ultimately develop the higher risk associated with their new country. Genetic factors are also important, however, as the natural history of breast cancer appears to vary between populations. In Japanese women, for example, the disease appears to develop earlier and to take a more benign course than in Western women. Also of striking significance is the rapid rise in incidence in some European countries, such as Spain, as their prosperity begins to approach that of the European Union as a whole.

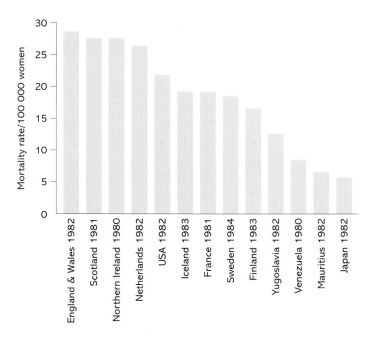

Figure 1.1 Breast cancer mortality rates show marked geographical variations.

In addition to age and geographical origin, numerous risk-modifying associations have been identified (Table 1.1).

Age

Age is by far the greatest risk factor for breast cancer (Figure 1.2). Of the approximately 60% of breast cancers for which identifiable risk factors can be found, age accounts for more than half.

Family history

The risk of breast cancer is increased 2–3-fold in women with a first-degree relative with breast cancer; the risk is also increased, but to a lesser extent, in women with a second-degree relative who is affected. The risk is particularly great if:

- the affected relative is on the maternal side of the family
- two first-degree relatives are affected
- the relative has bilateral breast cancer
- the relative's cancer was diagnosed before the age of 50 years.

TABLE 1.1

Factors influencing the risk of breast cancer

	High risk	Low risk
Relative risk 1.1–2.0		
Age at first full-term pregnancy	≥ 30	< 20
Age at menarche	< 12	> 14
Age at menopause	≥ 55	< 45
Obesity (postmenopausal)	Obese	Thin
Parity (postmenopausal)	Nulliparous	Multiparous
Breastfeeding (premenopausal)	None	Several years
Hormonal contraceptives	Yes	No
Hormone replacement therapy	Yes	No
Socioeconomic status	High	Low
Place of residence	Urban	Rural
Race/ethnicity		
Breast cancer at age < 40	Caucasian	Asian
Breast cancer at age ≥ 40	Black	Asian
Religion	Jewish	Mormon, Seventh-day Adventist
Relative risk 2.1–4.0		
Nodular densities on mammogram (postmenopausal)	> 75% of breast volume	Parenchyma composed entirely of fat
One first-degree relative with breast cancer	Yes	No
Biopsy-confirmed atypical hyperplasia	Yes	No
High-dose radiation to chest	Yes	No
Ovariectomy before age 35	No	Yes
Relative risk > 4.0		
Age	> 50	< 30
Country of birth	North America, Northern Europe	Asia, Africa
Two first-degree relatives with breast cancer diagnosed at an early age	Yes	No
History of cancer in one breast	Yes	No

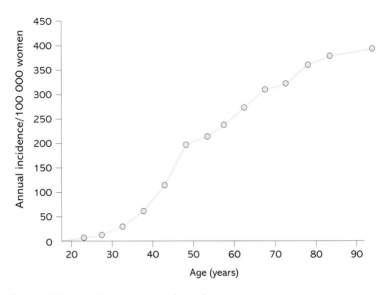

Figure 1.2 Age is the greatest risk factor for breast cancer.

Overall, about 10–15% of breast cancers are attributable to family history, and half of these can be attributed to specific susceptibility genes.

Demography
The risk of breast cancer is increased in women from higher socioeconomic classes, and in women living in urban areas.

Menses
The risk of breast cancer is increased in women who begin to menstruate at an early age (< 12 years) or who undergo the menopause at a relatively advanced age (> 55 years). Conversely, the risk is reduced in women in whom menarche is delayed, or who undergo bilateral ovariectomy before the age of about 35 years. This may partly explain the protective effect of early first pregnancy, as it has been suggested that it is the number of menstrual cycles before the first pregnancy that ultimately determines the risk of breast cancer. Thus, in Western countries with the highest incidences of breast cancer, menstruation typically begins at about the age of 12 years, but

the average age at first pregnancy is about 25 years. By contrast, in less developed countries, menstruation may not begin until the age of 17–18 years and the first pregnancy may have occurred by the age of 20 years.

Pregnancy

Age at first full-term pregnancy appears to be the most important factor in reducing the risk of breast cancer. For women who have their first child before the age of about 25 years, the risk of breast cancer is approximately half that for women who have their first child after 30 years of age, or who remain childless. Similarly, multiparous postmenopausal women have a lower risk of breast cancer than nulliparous women.

Some investigators have suggested the possibility that shortened pregnancy increases breast cancer risk. There are some animal models that support the hypothesis that early pregnancy stimulates proliferation of breast ductal tissue. This tissue only fully differentiates to genetically mature stable cells in late pregnancy. Thus, interrupting the cycle, either early (spontaneous or induced abortion) or late (prematurity), leaves a population of unstable cells. However, a large recent meta-analysis of 53 studies and 83 000 women in 16 countries largely refutes this hypothesis.

Obesity

Obesity is associated with an increased risk of breast cancer in postmenopausal women. This increased risk may be due to conversion of adrenal androgens to estrogens in adipose tissue.

High consumption of animal fats has also been linked to breast cancer. However, a recent meta-analysis of cohort studies involving over 330 000 women found no evidence for an association between the relative risk of breast cancer and dietary fat intake. Recent evidence from a study of the Chinese diet suggests that it is the high intake of phytoestrogens in vegetables and grains rather than low fat intake that exerts a protective effect. As a result, a clinical trial examining the effect of food additives derived from the oriental diet on the prevention of breast cancer has been proposed.

Oral contraceptives

A recent meta-analysis involving over 150 000 women has examined the influence of oral contraceptive (OC) use on the risk of breast cancer. The relative risk was slightly increased (1.24) in women who had used OCs within 10 years, but there was no excess risk in those who had used OCs more than 10 years previously. Although the incidence of breast cancer was increased in OC users, the disease mortality remained constant because the cancers tended to be of a more favorable type.

This slight increase in risk should, however, be viewed in the context of women's health in general. It is very likely that OCs substantially diminish the risk of ovarian and endometrial carcinoma. They are also highly effective as a form of contraception and as a means of relieving menses-related morbidity. There is no evidence that current formulations of OCs affect breast cancer risk. However, this will not be known for certain for another 30 years, since the cohort of women who have taken the pill (particularly low-dose preparations) are only now reaching the age at which they are at risk of breast cancer.

Hormone replacement therapy

The long-awaited results of a number of important trials have recently been published. To some extent these studies have confirmed and refined the risk of breast cancer associated with hormone replacement therapy (HRT), but many unanswered questions remain to be resolved. This complex issue is discussed fully in Chapter 7 (page 102).

Alcohol consumption

The consumption of approximately 15 g or more of alcohol (equivalent to 2–3 glasses of wine or measures of spirits) each day increases the risk of breast cancer by about 50%. This may be attributable to reduced hepatic estrogen metabolism. In practice, however, the increased risk associated with alcohol is small; it has been estimated that if 1000 women over 30 years of age maintained a moderate regular alcohol intake for 2 years one additional case of breast cancer might develop. This should be set against the potential reduction in ischemic heart disease associated with moderate alcohol consumption, and the contribution that alcohol could make to quality of life.

Genetics

With the rise of modern genetics research, a subcellular and molecular understanding of familial factors in breast cancer is emerging. New technologies have allowed detailed comparisons to be made between the chromosome patterns of 'normal' populations and those at high risk, which meant, initially, women with very strong family histories. From these studies, the first genes that were strongly associated with breast cancer were identified, notably *BRCA1* (17q21) and *BRCA2* (13q14). More recent research in Ashkenazi Jewish populations, in which the frequency of these genes is high, suggests that *BRCA1* and *BRCA2* are associated with a high risk of breast cancer, even in the absence of a family history. Furthermore, in the studied population, the risk effect is greater in those born after 1940 than in those born earlier. These genes are implicated in approximately 4% of all breast cancers and in up to 25% of patients diagnosed before the age of 40 years; they are also linked to ovarian cancers. The breast cancer risk associated with *BRCA2* appears less than that with *BRCA1*, but the presence of the gene mutation carries additional, smaller risks of male breast and prostate cancers, and perhaps others.

Neither *BRCA1* nor *BRCA2* should be considered 'breast-cancer specific' in the sense that a single mutation leads directly to disease, as in sickle-cell disease, for example. Both genes represent large segments on specific chromosomes where a number of deviations from the base sequence of DNA in the normal population are concentrated. It is believed that some of these changes result in inappropriate cellular proliferation, or are linked to a failure of DNA repair as a final common pathway. *BRCA1* does not appear to be a classic tumor suppressor gene, and somewhat paradoxically, it is not associated with sporadic cancers. However, there is some evidence that the gene may act in a novel way to suppress the function of other inhibitors of proliferation.

Normal *BRCA1* appears to suppress the signaling of mammary epithelial cells by the estrogen receptor. *BRCA2* is functionally related, but distinct. The BRCA proteins appear to play a subtle role in the central control of the sex steroid-regulated pathways, which is in keeping with the emerging understanding of cancer as a dynamic regulatory control disease. Whether these mutations predestine the cancer or merely facilitate malignant transformation is unknown. Recent data from twin studies suggest that these genes exert their influence very early, and set the context for the development of breast cancer in response to a hormonal stimulus that might otherwise be benign. Moreover, changes in *BRCA2* do not appear to be restricted to breast cancer. One of the genes closely associated with Fanconi's anemia appears to be identical to *BRCA2*. A fascinating postulate supported by early data is that *BRCA2* inherited from one parent leads to an elevated risk of breast and prostate cancer, but when inherited from both parents leads to a pediatric blood disorder.

BRCA1 and *BRCA2* are not the only genes implicated in breast cancer. One of the common DNA-sequence variants that confer a small increase in breast cancer risk is *CHEK2*. It is a component of the machinery that recognizes and repairs damaged DNA, and seems to activate *BRCA1*. Germline mutations in TP53 (p53 protein, Li–Fraumeni syndrome) usually lead to childhood cancers, but females who reach adulthood have a risk of breast cancer as high as 90%. *EMSY*, a newly identified gene, produces a protein that interacts with *BRCA2* and is overexpressed in sporadic breast cancers.

Although our understanding is rudimentary, a general concept emerges. Genes represent predisposition. The internal hormonal and regulatory milieu of the body, and life events such as diet, drugs, pregnancies and levels of activity are stimuli in a dynamic homeostatic process. The interaction between predisposition and provocation is when malignancy appears. It is reasonable to hypothesize that genes have an influence beyond susceptibility. Even in these early days, there is evidence that gene expression signatures can predict:

- risk of disease
- relapse and survival risk
- patterns of recurrence
- response to therapy.

When these regulatory pathways are better understood, establishing the point at which intervention is necessary will pose a substantial challenge and will profoundly influence our preventive and treatment strategies in the future.

Key points – epidemiology

- Age is the greatest risk factor.
- The breast cancer genes *BRCA1* and *BRCA2* denote high risk, but account for only a small proportion of cancers. Several other genes, including *CHEK2*, p53 and *EMSY*, are involved.
- Of the key factors, hormone replacement therapy is the most controversial (see Chapter 7).

Key references

Collaborative Group on Hormonal Factors in Breast Cancer. Breast cancer and hormonal contraceptives: collaborative reanalysis of individual data on 53 297 women with breast cancer and 100 239 women without breast cancer from 54 epidemiological studies. *Lancet* 1996;347:1713–27.

Collaborative Group on Hormonal Factors in Breast Cancer. Breast cancer and abortion: collaborative reanalysis of data from 53 epidemiological studies, including 83 000 women with breast cancer from 16 countries. *Lancet* 2004;363: 1007–16.

Hughes-Davis L, Huntsman D, Ruas M et al. EMSY links the *BRCA2* pathway to sporadic breast and ovarian cancer. *Cell* 2003;115: 523–35.

Kelsey JL. A review of the epidemiology of human breast cancer. *Epidemiol Rev* 1979;1: 74–109.

Levi F, Luchini F, Negri E, La Vecchia C. The fall in breast cancer mortality in Europe. *Eur J Cancer* 2001;37:1409–12.

Neiburgs H. Molecular genetics and cancer: the role of *BRCA1* and *BRCA2*. *Womens Oncol Rev* 2002;2:19–29.

Saunders CM, Baum M. Breast cancer and pregnancy: a review. *J R Soc Med* 1993;86:162–5.

Special news report. Epidemiology faces its limits. *Science* 1995;269: 164–9.

Thompson WD. Genetic epidemiology of breast cancer. *Cancer* 1994;74(suppl):279–87.

Van de Vijver MJ, He YD, van't Veer LJ et al. A gene-expression signature as a predictor of survival in breast cancer. *N Engl J Med* 2002; 347:1999–2009.

Wooster R, Weber BL. Breast and ovarian cancer. *N Engl J Med* 2003;348:2339–47.

Despite current preoccupation with the notion of risk, it is a poorly understood concept, and even more questionably acted on in public policy and healthcare. Breast cancer in all its aspects is under intense scrutiny, and three areas in particular are controversial: screening, adjuvant therapy and the treatment of advanced disease. Moreover, the clinical trials process, which is essential to increasing our understanding of cancer, is all about risk.

Three definitions form the basis of risk assessment:

- risk or odds
- consequence or harm
- balance or comparison.

Risk is a measurement of likelihood, or how often an event takes place. It is a proportional quantity. Implicit in the concept is a comparison of the number of times an event might occur with the number of times it actually does occur. For example, if the risk of falling off a mountain is estimated to be 1/10 000, then for every 10 000 individual mountain-climbing excursions, one person falls. The term 'risk' carries a negative connotation, though in fact it is intended to be a neutral term; conversely 'odds' has a more positive implication (e.g. the odds of winning).

In general, it is not possible to reduce the risk of an event to zero, and the effort required to reach the asymptote becomes disproportionate. Moreover, it is not necessary to do something in order to encounter risk, because doing nothing can also engender risk. A specific risk is always in competition with another risk, the outcome of which will depend partly on the path chosen and how carefully risk events are identified. If you choose to drive 1000 miles because of fear of flying, the risk shift introduces direct road hazards, loss of time, the joy of seeing the countryside go by and, ultimately, the possibility that a crashing plane might land on top of you!

Relative risk. Calculating risk becomes more difficult as an event becomes rarer and when complex interdependent events are considered.

The notion of relative risk arises when the same event can take place whatever course of action is chosen. Sometimes the same event can result from different causes. To continue the example, whether you die in a plane crash or by the roadside, you are still dead. Where it is possible to assign cause to the event, it is called a cause-specific risk. This can be very difficult to determine, because events have multiple causes; for example, death while flying might have had nothing to do with being in the plane and could have been due to an intracerebral bleed. Finally, it is not possible to anticipate or identify all possible risks, which is sometimes referred to as the law of unintended consequences (that is, actions always have effects that are unanticipated or unintended).

Consequence or harm represents the severity of the effect of the risk event should it happen, which also carries a negative connotation. The total effect of a given risk is the product of the risk and the consequence. Numerous studies have shown that people tend to pay more attention to negative consequences than positive ones, particularly when the former are seen as gruesome, refractory to treatment and poorly understood.

There is an important corollary to the notion that no risk exists in isolation. Conceptually, the proper approach to the assessment of risk would be to sum the product of all possible risks and their consequences. In reality, this is very difficult to do and, as a result, there is often an exaggerated focus on rare, potentially dramatic adverse consequences.

Balance or comparison is another vital principle. The concept of relative or proportionate risk underlies all of medicine. When considering individual hazards, it is important to make the distinction between the proportionate risk (i.e. the ratio of events taking place with or without intervention) and the absolute risk (i.e. the likelihood of the event as a proportion of the entire population at risk). A small proportionate advance against a high-frequency risk may be of greater consequence than a large advance against a rare risk. This issue becomes significant in discussions about adjuvant therapy for breast cancer.

Explaining the concept of risk

People have some sense of the total effect of a specific risk. However, there is no metric for identifying, summing and weighing all hazards and consequences. The event risks are constantly changing. The consequences vary with time and circumstance, and individuals making personal choices change their internal evaluation strategies over time. The best approach is to give a clear explanation of the basic principles and to set individual risk/consequence discussions in the context of the other hazards that exist. There is no single risk that exists in isolation.

Thus, when explaining the concept of risk to a patient, there are a number of points worth considering.

- It is helpful to set risk in context, by comparing the risk of breast cancer with that of trauma or heart disease.
- The distinction between risk and consequence should be clarified.
- Risk is a proportional quantity. A doubling of a very small risk may be far less worrisome than a 5% increase in a very large risk.
- All interventions, including doing nothing, involve a trade-off of risks.

Screening

Breast cancer screening, for an individual woman, is an exercise in understanding the basic principle of risk – the likelihood of an adverse event. Women generally grossly overestimate their risk of developing breast cancer and, as a consequence, overrate the benefits that may be gained from screening. A recent study of well-educated women in the USA found that they overestimated their risk of dying from breast cancer in the next 10 years by an average of 22 times (range 17–58 times) and overrated the absolute benefits of screening by 127 times (range 99–299 times). It is important, therefore, that women are educated about the concept of risk and the terms used to describe it, in order that they may make informed choices with regard to screening and treatment. Figure 2.1 depicts the effect of breast screening in 1000 women aged 50 over the subsequent 25 years, and shows that a relatively large relative risk reduction translates into a relatively small change in absolute benefit.

Describing the risk of developing breast cancer as 1 in 10–12 is true, yet unhelpful, because this figure is the cumulative risk for those

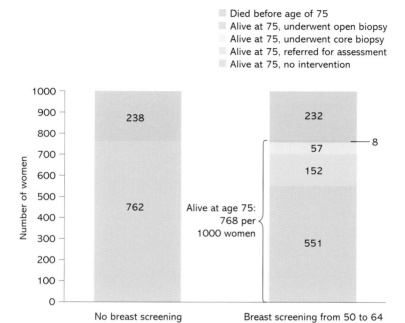

Figure 2.1 The effect of breast screening on outcome. Figure reproduced with permission from Marshall T, Adab P. Informed consent for breast screening: what should we tell women? *J Med Screen* 2003;10:22–6.

women who live to be 85 years old. In real terms, the background risk for women between the ages of 30 and 50 is about 1/1000/year or 2% on aggregate, whereas before the age of 30 breast cancer is exceptionally rare. Between the ages of 50 and 70, the time during which mammographic screening is most often recommended, the risk goes up to about 2/1000/year, which is approximately 2% on aggregate in the first decade of the menopause, rising steeply thereafter, with about one-third of all reported breast cancers occurring in the extreme age group of 70–85 years.

All the excess relative risks, apart from a very strong family history or previous biopsy of atypical hyperplasia, are less than 2 – in other words, less than a doubling of the background risk. It is also important to note that the observational data from which these relative risks are calculated have methodological weaknesses, and leading statisticians have questioned whether a relative risk below 2 is not within the experimental error of the method.

It is important to explain what any increase in relative risk means in real terms. For example, if a woman finds out that she has a relative risk of breast cancer that is twice that of the normal population, she may understandably panic and assume that she has a 1 in 6 chance of dying of the disease within the foreseeable future. Yet if she is 30 years old her risk doubles to 2/1000/year or 2% in a decade, which might seem insignificant against the other risks of living in a modern urban society. Furthermore, any increases in the relative risks are not distributed symmetrically throughout a woman's lifetime, but tend to occur by the age of 60, after which the risk levels return to normal. Women counseled in this way are often comforted and do not feel the need for unnecessary mammographic screening, and are unlikely to contemplate prophylactic mastectomy, which is a growth industry in the USA.

The identification of some breast cancer genes (*BRCA1*, *BRCA2*) among women with a poor family history is, of course, a different matter altogether. These women have a 50/50 chance of inheriting the gene. Early data suggested that the breast cancer risk of women who carried the gene might be as high as 85%, but more recent data from Europe seem to indicate that the risk is of the order of 50%. The potential advantage of genetic testing in women with very strong family histories is that a negative result would effectively reduce the woman's risk to the level in the background population, and thus alleviate much concern and perhaps unnecessary intervention. On the other hand, a positive result might lead to more rational decisions about prophylactic mastectomy.

There are several analytic tables and software programs that extrapolate from epidemiological databases to estimate individual risk. The Claus model uses empirical data from the Cancer and Steroid Hormone Study. It is constructed on the principle that inherited risk is attributable to a rare autosomal-dominant mutation with high penetrance. The estimate is based on a woman's age, the number of first- and second-degree relatives with breast cancer, and their age at the onset of the disease. There is some likelihood of underestimation as other factors are not considered. The Gale model uses data from the Breast Cancer Demonstration Detection Project. In contrast to the Claus model, the focus is on the patient and first-degree relatives, and so this model may overestimate the risk in those with close relatives with breast cancer and underestimate the risk for others. The tables are complex, but compact software has been developed which makes the model more accessible.

Chemoprevention of breast cancer with tamoxifen

In 1985, Cuzick and Baum were the first to report that patients treated with adjuvant tamoxifen had a significant reduction in the risk of contralateral breast cancer. Since then, a number of large multicenter trials have investigated the potential of tamoxifen to prevent breast cancer in high-risk women. The International Breast Cancer Intervention Study (IBIS) in the UK and Australia began first, but was rapidly overtaken by phase 1 of the North American National Surgical Adjuvant Breast and Bowel Project NSABP(P1), which reported a significant reduction in the incidence of new breast cancers in women exposed to tamoxifen. In absolute terms, this trial found that 6000 well women treated with tamoxifen for 5 years experienced a delay in the appearance of 80 estrogen-receptor-positive (ER+ve) cases of breast cancer.

Despite publication of this report, the IBIS trial continued recruiting and reported their results last year, together with an overview of the four tamoxifen prevention trials (NSABP[P1], IBIS, Milan and Royal Marsden). Again, the tamoxifen group demonstrated a significant reduction in the incidence of ER+ve breast cancers. However, an excess of endometrial cancers and a significant excess of deaths from thromboembolic events occurred. As a result of an excess of deaths from non-breast cancer causes, the overall mortality in the tamoxifen and placebo groups remained the same but, of course, there were more adverse events in the treated arm. For these reasons, there is no transatlantic consensus, and the European point of view would be to consider tamoxifen prevention still experimental. This case is a perfect example of the notion of competing risks or the law of unintended consequences.

Meanwhile, a new and very large trial in the USA to compare tamoxifen with raloxifene (a new selective estrogen-receptor modulator) is rapidly recruiting. The trial will at least balance the undoubted benefits of raloxifene in preventing osteoporosis against the potential of the two compounds for delaying or preventing the appearance of breast cancer, and the risk with tamoxifen of inducing endometrial cancer or venous thromboembolic disease.

Treatment of early breast cancer

Proportional risk is perhaps the most important concept to arise from the many trials of systemic (adjuvant) therapy for early breast cancer. Each type of treatment reduces the risk of breast cancer recurrence by a relatively constant proportion. Thus, in premenopausal women, chemotherapy reduces the risk of recurrence by 33% and ovariectomy by about 25%, while in postmenopausal women, tamoxifen reduces the risk by about 40%. Thus, the benefit for a given woman in absolute terms depends on both the effect of treatment on the relative risk and underlying individual risk factors. Fundamental to interpreting estimates of benefit is the understanding that the proportion being calculated relates to the number of adverse events, not the number of persons at risk. For example, a premenopausal woman with a 1.5 cm tumor without nodal involvement may have a 10-year risk of recurrence of 10% (1 in 10). If adjuvant chemotherapy produces a relative risk reduction of about 30% then, in absolute terms, the patient gains 30% of 10% in the chance of living disease-free for 10 years, or a gain of about 3%. On the other hand, if the same woman has four nodes involved, her 10-year risk of recurrence is about 50%. The treatment offers a 30% relative risk reduction, leading to an absolute benefit of 30% of 50%, or a 15% decrease in the probability of recurrence within 10 years.

There are two important further considerations. First, the data from which these recommendations derive are generally specific for the risk of breast cancer; competing adverse risks, including the toxicity of treatment, are not considered. In that respect, the data may overestimate benefit. Secondly, in contrast to the benefit being calculated against the number of adverse events, the toxicity of treatment affects the entire population treated and not solely those who experience an adverse event. Thus, if the risk of an adverse event is 25%, then 1 in 4 of those who receive the treatment will experience the effect. If only 3 in 100 benefit from a reduction in the recurrence risk, it might be said that 25 people experience side effects in order that 3 accrue a benefit. Clearly, the greater the recurrence risk, the more likely people will be willing to accept toxicity. These are complex issues which cannot be discussed fully in this limited overview. Figure 2.2 (pages 24–5) provides some clarification of the central concepts relating to the risks and benefits of treatment, and new computer software is now available to help women make informed choices in selecting adjuvant systemic therapy based on this principle.

Advanced disease

At present, treatment of recurrent or advanced disease is not likely to extend survival in most patients. The risk discussion thus becomes one of comparing and contrasting consequences. In this setting, the baseline consequences are symptoms or closely anticipated symptoms, and the consequence of intervention is side effects. The risk-management strategy becomes one of direct trade-off, namely 'paying' for a diminution of disease-related morbidity with treatment-related morbidity. In some respects the calculation is more difficult, since the 'event' being sought is not discrete (as in a recurrence), but an alteration in symptoms or signs.

Key points – perception of risk

- Risk is a poorly understood concept – nothing is risk-free.
- Risk measures the likelihood that an event will take place.
- Risk is a proportional quantity.
- Consequence represents the severity of effect of an event.
- Decision-making involves balancing of risks.
- Correct decisions about lifestyle choices, screening and selection of adjuvant systemic therapy depend on the understanding of these issues.

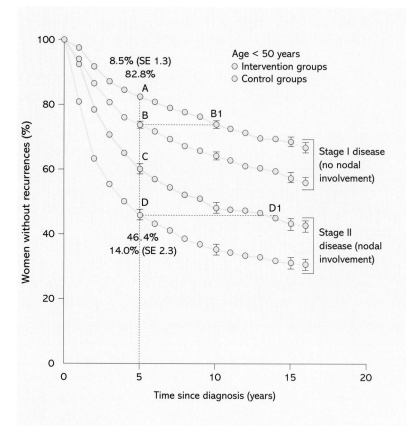

Figure 2.2 This figure is intended to clarify concepts relating to the risks and benefits of treatment for early stage breast cancer. The figure is derived from the Early Breast Cancer Trialists' Collaborative Group Overview, and is intended as an example.

The two upper curves represent women without nodal involvement (Stage I). The lower pair represents those with evidence of nodal involvement. In both pairs, the upper curve is the intervention arm, the lower the control arm. The plots are arithmetic, though these data are often presented in semilogarithmic form.

For this example, consider the results at 5 years. The issue is the number of 'events', meaning recurrences, which have been prevented or delayed at this point.

Figure 2.2 continued

For stage I women, point **B** is the proportion of women whose tumors recurred without treatment, 25.8% (100 − 74.2). Point **A** is the proportion who had recurrences despite treatment, 17.2% (100 − 82.8). The risk reduction can be presented two ways:

- as a proportion of those whose tumors recurred without treatment, calculated as (25.8 − 17.2)/25.8 = 0.3333 or 33.3%
- as a proportion of the treatment population, sometimes called the absolute benefit, calculated as the risk without treatment minus the risk with treatment, in this case 82.8 − 74.2 = 8.6%.

For stage II women, the calculations are as follows. Point **C** represents recurrence in women receiving treatment, 39.6% (100 − 60.4), and point **D** the recurrence rate in the control arm, 53.6% (100 − 46.4). Again, the risk reduction can be presented two ways:

- as a proportion of those whose tumors recurred without treatment, calculated as (53.6 − 39.6)/53.6 = 0.261 or 26.1%
- as the absolute benefit, in this case 53.6 − 39.6 = 14%.

The crucial message is the distinction between proportionate and absolute benefit. In this case, the proportionate benefit for intervention in stage I disease appears greater than that in stage II (33.3 % vs 26.1%). However, in absolute terms, stage II patients derive a greater benefit (14% vs 8.6%). The explanation is that there are more recurrences to start with in stage II disease.

Finally, the horizontal distances B to B1 and D to D1 are occasionally used to estimate the 'time gained' by virtue of the treatment. This is a controversial analysis, in part because it assumes that those patients who have recurrences are otherwise biologically identical to those who do not, and that the difference is solely due to treatment. Given that there are significant numbers of women whose cancers would not have recurred, even without intervention, that assumption may not be entirely true.

Key references

Becher H, Chang-Claude J. Estimating disease risks for individuals with a given family history in different populations with an application to breast cancer. *Genet Epidemiol* 1996;13:229–42.

Benichou J, Gale MH, Mulvihill JJ. Graphs to estimate an individualized risk of breast cancer. *J Clin Oncol* 1996;14:103–10.

Bianchi S, Palli D, Galli M, Zampi G. Benign breast disease and cancer risk. *Crit Rev Oncol Hematol* 1993; 15:221–42.

Black WC, Nease RF, Tosteson AVA. Perceptions of breast cancer risk and screening effectiveness in women younger than 50 years of age. *J Natl Cancer Inst* 1995;87:720–3.

Claus EB, Risch N, Thompson WD. Autosomal dominant inheritance of early-onset breast cancer. Implications for risk prediction. *Cancer* 1994;73:643–51.

Colditz GA, Hankinson SE, Hunter DJ et al. The use of estrogens and progestins and the risk of breast cancer in post-menopausal women. *N Engl J Med* 1995;332:1589–93.

Cuzick J, Powles T, Veronesi U et al. Overview of the main outcomes in breast-cancer prevention trials. *Lancet* 2003;361:296–300.

Dupont WD, Page DL. Risk factors for breast cancer in women with proliferative disease. *N Engl J Med* 1985;312:146–51.

Fisher B, Costantino JP, Redmond CK et al. Endometrial cancer in tamoxifen-treated breast cancer patients: findings from the National Surgical Adjuvant Breast and Bowel Project (NSABP) B-14. *J Natl Cancer Inst* 1994;86:527–37.

Hulka BS, Stark AT. Breast cancer: cause and prevention. *Lancet* 1995; 346:883–7.

Jatoi I, Baum M. American and European recommendations for screening mammography in younger women: a cultural divide? *BMJ* 1993;307:1481–3.

Kopans DB. Screening for breast cancer and mortality reduction among women 40–49 years of age. *Cancer* 1994;74:311–22.

Madigan MP, Ziegler RG, Benichou J et al. Proportion of breast cancer cases in the United States explained by well-established risk factors. *J Natl Cancer Inst* 1995;87:1681–5.

NHS Breast Screening Programme 1996 Review. The Manor House, 260 Eccles Hall Road South, Sheffield.

Whitehead MI, Godfree V. *HRT, your questions answered*. London: Churchill Livingstone, 1992:89–99.

The biological enigma

Breast cancer is an enigmatic disease. Although it is possible to make broad generalizations about risk, natural history and clinical pattern, the future for any individual woman (and the occasional man) who develops breast cancer is highly unpredictable. Consider the following observations.

- The risk of breast cancer begins at puberty and rises slowly until the perimenopausal years, when it increases dramatically, eventually leveling off at about the age of 75 years. Women who do not achieve menses seldom get breast cancer. Apart from aging, which is by far the largest risk factor, the lifetime exposure to menstrual cycles, and particularly age at onset of menses, is the most important non-genetic risk factor.

- Breast cancer stage appears to be a biological property of the tumor rather than simply an expression of anatomical spread. The natural history of breast cancer is determined by the stage at diagnosis; thus, the risk of recurrence of a stage II tumor is inherently worse than that of a stage I tumor. Moreover, irrespective of grade or stage, the risk of recurrence peaks at about 3 years, then flattens for a few years, with a second unexplained peak appearing between 7 and 10 years, before settling down to a constant hazard for the rest of the patient's life (breast cancers detected early by mammography may prove to be an exception).

- Highly aggressive surgical procedures are no better than limited excision for local and systemic management of breast cancer.

- When breast cancer recurs, it can show a variety of presentations, depending on the time to relapse and the site of tissue recurrence. For example, the longer the disease-free interval, the better the prognosis and the more likely the tumor is to be ER+ve or progesterone-receptor positive (PR+ve) and to have metastasized to bone.

- The anatomical distribution of the disease shows several curious clusters. In some cases, the tumor may be locally aggressive (particularly on the chest wall) and refractory to therapy, yet show little propensity to wider dissemination until much later. Bony metastases can wax and wane for years. Occasionally, the disease is explosive in both time and distribution, mimicking an infectious process. Histopathologically, the outcome cannot be predicted from the original tissue.

- Hormone manipulation is more effective in postmenopausal women than in younger women. For cytotoxic therapies, however, the opposite is true.

Breast biology

To appreciate the significance of these observations, it is helpful to consider the development of the human breast and breast cancer as a biological process.

The breast is an epithelial organ that develops in the embryo from the ectodermal primitive milk streak, or 'galactic band'. This ridge of tissue extends from the axilla to the groin, and is responsible for the supernumerary breasts occasionally seen in humans, and familiar in other mammalian species. The breast parenchyma is thought to develop from sweat glands, and is independent of hormonal influence during this early stage. By the third trimester of pregnancy, placental sex hormones enter the fetal circulation and induce canalization of early branched epithelial tissues. The 'witch's milk' that may occur in neonates of both sexes is secreted from these early glands.

The breast then remains relatively quiescent until puberty when, under the influence of hypothalamic gonadotropin-releasing hormones, primordial ovarian follicles mature and produce estrogens that stimulate the growth and maturation of breast and other sensitive tissues. With the onset of ovulatory menstrual cycles, the breast begins a period of cyclic stimulation and regression that continues until interrupted by pregnancy, the menopause or certain pharmacological and other interventions, such as intensive physical training.

Breast cancer. It is, perhaps, a truism to suggest that breast cancer is the result of a subtle imbalance in the complex regulatory cycles to which breast tissue is exposed. Sex hormones, epidermal growth factors

(EGFs) and other agents that influence normal growth and function do so by up- and downregulating genetic pathways leading to cell proliferation and regression. The induction and promotion of breast cancer is a multifactorial and multistep process, in which a series of defenses must be overcome over a period of time, though not necessarily in a rigidly defined order. As this process develops from an early genetic predisposition, each defect in the regulatory system contributes to a cascade. In time, and in the face of numerous external stimuli, the family of defects expands, eventually leading to cellular immortalization and the molecular expression of the drivers of the classic malignant triad of growth, invasion and metastasis (Figure 3.1).

The subtle dividing line between benign and malignant changes is seen in ductal carcinoma in situ. There is now evidence that, in this situation, tumor sensitivity to growth hormones is increased, but the tumor lacks the abnormal ability to traverse the basement membrane, and thus may reach a considerable size yet remain localized. The subsequent emergence of the ability of the tumor to cross the basement membrane, apparently characterized by the production of specific gene products such as hyaluronidase, heralds invasion and increased risk of systemic disease. It is likely that each step in the triad of growth, invasion and metastasis is controlled by specific proteins secreted by the tumor or surrounding tissue. Thus, while the tissues from different patients may have the same histopathological appearance, the genetic and metabolic machinery will differ. The mixture of defects involved is likely to determine the clinical pattern of the disease.

Viewing the breast as a complex organ in which subtle, and perhaps cumulative, small defects after each menstrual cycle lead to an overall failure of regulation may put the disease process into context. Breast cancer is age-related because multiple defects are involved; the clinical stage and pattern of disease are functions of these defects. Moreover, there is a dynamic relationship between the tumor and the host, and thus the defects are themselves in constant flux. Patterns of incidence and recurrence seem to parallel known major changes in the regulatory milieu, such as the menopause and possibly other, as yet uncharacterized, events.

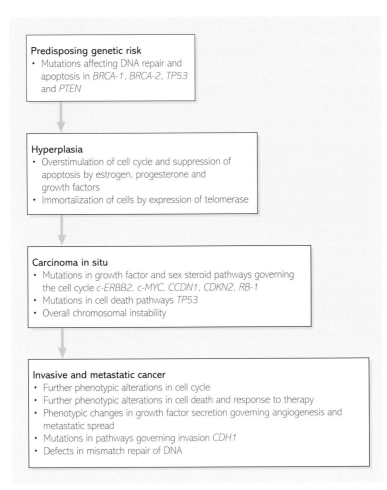

Figure 3.1 The genetic and phenotypic changes in mammary epithelial cells associated with the onset and progression of breast cancer.

Though the notion of cancer as an abnormal growth goes back thousands of years, modern understanding dates from the advent of light microscopy and histopathological preparation methods. Early pathologists were struck by the apparent progressive cellular and organic disorganization of tumors. Early prognostic indicators were predominantly measures of disorganization – differentiation in pathological terms. The triad of uncontrolled growth, invasion and metastasis served then, as now, as the descriptive hallmark of cancer.

It is also of historical note that the same microscopic techniques led to the observation of microbial infectious disease and, with that conceptual development, the notion of disease as a foreign invader requiring eradication. That notion has served as the basis of successful anti-infective therapies and, until recently, also as the basis of cancer treatment.

However, cancer is different. In the first instance, it is a process which, once initiated, is a disease of host tissue. Moreover, in recent years, understanding at the molecular and tissue levels has evolved such that malignancy is now seen as the result of a multistep induction process that never reaches an endpoint. It is a constantly evolving dynamic in which communities of cells lose their organizational discipline. It is genetically driven, by both spontaneous and internally and externally driven changes in the genes of individual cells, which result in altered regulatory processes governing the day-to-day life of the cell (Figure 3.2).

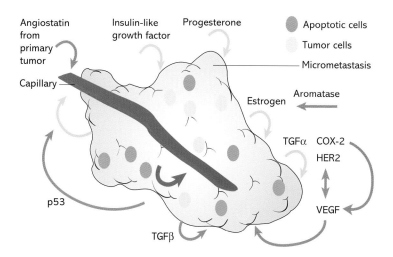

Figure 3.2 A schematic illustration of a hypothetical micrometastasis. The tumor is in a state of dynamic equilibrium as a result of its microenvironment, a 'soup' of cytokines; these cytokines balance angiogenesis, epithelial proliferation and apoptosis. Surgery might unbalance this equilibrium and 'kick-start' active growth, leading to the first peak incidence of clinically obvious secondaries within two years.

31

Cancer cells were previously thought to be truly autonomous from their surroundings, but this is now known to be untrue. Cancer cells interact intensely with their surroundings; it is the signaling that is misguided. Paradoxically, cancer cells are often overly sensitive to otherwise appropriate stimuli. Moreover, cancer as a process extends beyond the cancer cell. The real action is at the interface between what are perceived to be the cancer cells and the ostensibly normal tissues adjacent to those cells.

More than 95% of breast cancers are epithelial tumors, arising from either the milk-producing glands (lobular carcinoma) or the draining ducts (ductal carcinoma). As an endocrine-related tumor, breast cancer shares with prostate, thyroid and other rarer epithelial malignancies an enigmatic, time-variable history quite distinct from other common epithelial tumors such as those derived from the colon and lung. The patterns of long disease-free intervals followed by cyclic recurrence and remission are characteristic of these endocrine-related epithelial malignancies. The natural history of colon cancer, viewed from a population perspective, has a flat tail of long-term survivors, apparently cured. Breast cancer is fundamentally different (Figure 3.3). The survival curve never flattens. The risk of recurrence, on a proportionate basis, remains constant for life and is determined by the initial stage of the tumor. Moreover, there have been observations of periods of somewhat increased recurrence risk 2–3 years after diagnosis. All of this suggests a very subtle regulatory process that has both spontaneous and therapy-associated perturbations. This has caused renewed controversy in the clinical and research literature about whether some or all of the benefits of adjuvant chemotherapy really reflect hormonal manipulation by another means, and whether the act of surgery 'kick-starts' the dormant metastases by inducing angiogenesis.

The current treatment guidelines presented in *Fast Facts – Breast Cancer* have been derived from a classical model of the disease, which is now evolving rapidly. As breast cancer is more fully understood as a systemic regulatory disease with events at the time of surgery critical for outcome, treatment strategies will change, and perhaps the enigma will begin to dissipate.

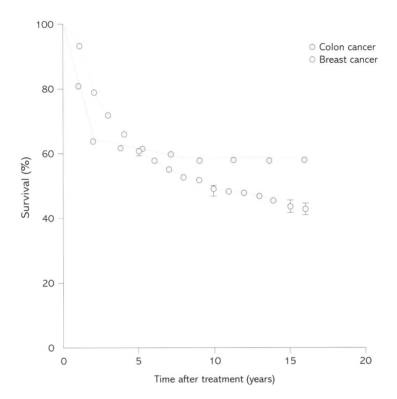

Figure 3.3 Comparison of survival in breast and colon cancer. In colon cancer, there is a flat tail on the survival curve after about 5 years and, in the absence of a second malignancy, these patients can be considered 'cured'. The breast cancer curve, however, does not exhibit such a tail. This biological difference underlies current treatment strategies and also offers insights into why the benefits of breast cancer interventions are likely to take longer to ascertain than those for colon cancer.

Structure of the breast and surrounding tissues

The breast is composed of glandular and adipose tissue in varying proportions. The glandular tissue consists of 15–20 lobes containing numerous lobules, linked by ductules (Figure 3.4). The ductules combine to form the lactiferous ducts, which open into the lactiferous sinuses and empty through the nipple. The breast is enclosed in two layers of fibrous tissue – a superficial layer and a thicker deep layer overlying the chest muscles; the two layers are connected by Cooper's ligaments (Figure 3.4).

The principal muscles related to the breast are:
- the pectoralis major
- the pectoralis minor
- the serratus anterior
- the latissimus dorsi.

The blood supply to the breast has two main components. The outer region of the breast is supplied by branches of the axillary artery, whereas the inner region is supplied by arteries arising from the internal mammary artery. Similarly, lymph from the outer region drains into the axillary lymph nodes, while lymph from the inner region is drained via the lymph nodes associated with the internal mammary artery.

Benign breast disease

Although a lump in the breast is the first symptom in 80–90% of cases of breast cancer, about 80% of breast lumps are due to benign breast disease. The most common causes of benign breast disease are listed in Table 3.1.

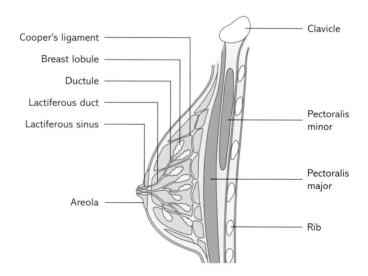

Cooper's ligament

Breast lobule

Ductule

Lactiferous duct

Lactiferous sinus

Areola

Clavicle

Pectoralis minor

Pectoralis major

Rib

Figure 3.4 Structure of the normal breast.

TABLE 3.1

Classification of benign breast disease

Benign neoplasia

- Fibroadenoma
- Lipoma
- Duct papilloma
- Skin lesions

Dysplasia

- Abnormalities of normal development and involution (nodularity)
- Solitary cysts
- Epithelial hyperplasia/atypia

Trauma

- Hematoma
- Fat necrosis

Inflammatory disease

- Puerperal abscess
- Periductal (plasma cell) mastitis
- Tuberculosis

Developmental

- Supernumerary breast
- Absent breast
- Asymmetrical breast development

Benign breast disease is the most common cause of breast problems, and affects up to 30% of women. Fibroadenomas and diffuse nodularity are most common in young women (< 30 years of age), whereas cysts are most common over the age of 40 years (Figure 3.5).

Solitary cysts are among the most common benign breast tumors in women aged 35–55 years. They can be diagnosed and treated by needle aspiration of the cyst contents.

Fibroadenomas account for 13% of all breast tumors, and are most common in women below 30 years of age, in whom they account for 60% of palpable lumps. Fewer than 10% of fibroadenomas increase in size, and approximately one-third decrease in size or disappear. Fibroadenomas over 4 cm in diameter should be excised. Smaller tumors do not need to be excised in women under 30 years of age if the diagnosis has been confirmed by cytology, but excision is appropriate in older women to avoid the risk of overlooking breast cancer.

Epithelial dysplasia may be a chance finding following biopsy of a 'lumpy breast'. The combination of epithelial hyperplasia and cellular atypia is termed atypical hyperplasia, and is a potentially premalignant condition; the 10-year risk of breast cancer if atypical hyperplasia is present is 8% for a woman without a first-degree relative with breast cancer, and 20–25% for a woman with an affected first-degree relative.

Breast cancer

Most malignant breast tumors originate in the epithelia of the terminal ducts and lobules; only a small number involve the stroma or soft tissues. The most common classification describes tumors on the basis

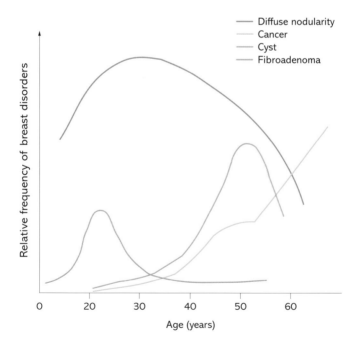

Figure 3.5 Fibroadenomas and diffuse nodularity are most common in women aged less than 30 years. By contrast, benign cysts and breast cancer become more common above the age of 40 years.

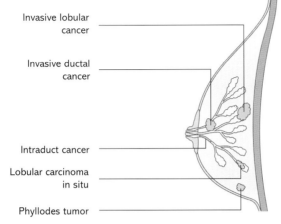

Invasive lobular cancer

Invasive ductal cancer

Intraduct cancer

Lobular carcinoma in situ

Phyllodes tumor

Figure 3.6 Types of breast cancer.

of their origins (ducts or lobules) and according to whether they are confined to their original site or have invaded surrounding tissues (Figure 3.6). There is emerging evidence that, like hematopoietic tissues, solid organs, including the breast, retain primordial stem cells. Regulatory defects in these cells have been identified, and may serve as the nidus of malignancy. If so, our diagnostic and treatment strategies will have to evolve again.

Histologically, breast cancers are characterized by groups of abnormal cells in a matrix of normal fibrous tissue. The degree of differentiation can be expressed according to the Scarf, Bloom and Richardson scale, in which glandular formation, nuclear pleomorphism and frequency of mitoses are each scored from 1 to 3. Highly differentiated tumors (grade I, score 3–5) are associated with a better prognosis than poorly differentiated tumors (grade III, score 8–9; Figure 3.7).

Invasive ductal carcinomas account for over 90% of breast cancers. They generally present as a hard, poorly defined lump. Involvement of the ligaments and ducts leads to dimpling and pitting of the skin, and nipple inversion (Figure 3.8).

Invasive lobular carcinoma is responsible for approximately 8% of breast cancers. Such tumors may occur at several sites, either in the same breast or in both breasts. The physical signs and characteristics of lobular

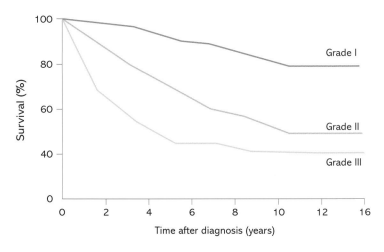

Figure 3.7 Useful prognostic information can be obtained from the degree of tumor differentiation. Highly differentiated tumors (grade I) are associated with markedly improved survival compared with less well-differentiated tumors (grades II and III).

cancers may be similar to those of ductal cancer, but are often hard to diagnose because of their diffuse nature and relative radiolucency, which means that they often do not show up on mammograms.

Phyllodes tumors (cystosarcoma phyllodes) are relatively rare stromal tumors. They do occasionally show cystic degeneration, but only very rarely exhibit the malignant features of a true sarcoma. Clinically and on imaging, they resemble fibroadenomas, although they are often larger than 2 cm in diameter. Microscopically the epithelial elements are normal, but the stromal areas show abnormal numbers of fibroblasts, some of which have a primitive morphology. They are subdivided into low-grade (the majority) and high-grade (about 5%). Low-grade tumors may be treated in the same manner as fibroadenomas, and high-grade tumors as for sarcoma with radical excision. Like other stromal maligancies, these tumors tend to metastasize to the lung.

Preinvasive carcinomas are referred to as ductal carcinomas or lobular carcinomas in situ (DCIS or LCIS, respectively). Lumps are seldom

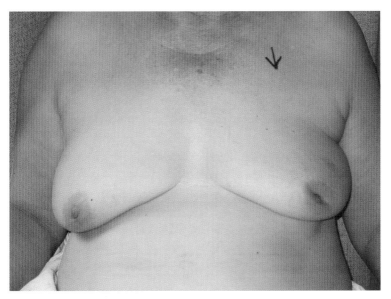

Figure 3.8 Clinical appearance of an invasive ductal carcinoma in the left breast of an elderly woman. Note the appearance of the nipple.

detectable, and most such tumors are detected by mammographic screening of the breast or as chance findings after a biopsy of a benign lesion. The proportion of in-situ carcinomas that progress to invasive disease is unknown, though postmortem studies suggest that it may be as low as 20%. The risk of invasive cancer is believed to be increased about elevenfold in a woman in whom DCIS is treated by removal of the affected area alone.

Natural history of breast cancer

At one extreme, women may present with massive involvement of the axillary nodes or even bone-marrow infiltration, with the primary tumor virtually undetectable, and die of breast cancer before the primary disease is clinically apparent. At the other extreme, women may refuse treatment and live for 20–30 years with a slowly progressive cancer which, though it may present an unpleasant problem for the patient, seems to lack the capacity to metastasize and kill. Furthermore, following apparently successful treatment, women can relapse and die up to 20–30 years after the initial diagnosis. It is also curious that, irrespective of the disease-free interval between diagnosis and relapse, the subsequent behavior of the disease becomes predictable. No patients have been cured once distant relapse has been diagnosed, and the median expectation of survival is about 2 years, though the range is wide. Certainly, those patients with a longer disease-free interval are more likely to respond to endocrine treatments which, in rare cases, are associated with prolonged remission.

Of particular note is the aggressive nature of breast cancer in very young women; for those under the age of 34 years at diagnosis, less than half can be expected to survive 5 years, with most relapsing within the first 3 years after treatment. Another curiosity yet to be explained adequately is the prognostic significance of chest wall recurrence. A patient may have a perfectly adequate mastectomy with wide margins of clearance on pathological assessment, but subsequently develop a crop of nodules on the chest wall, which are recurrent breast cancer, followed within a short interval by distant metastases, leading to death.

Staging of breast cancer

Accurate clinical staging for breast cancer has always been considered essential as a guide to prognosis and treatment. It defines the limits of primary surgical approaches (to Stage I and 2), and establishes the prognostic setting for radiation and systemic treatments. The original reason for this was the recognition, back in the early 1940s, that many of the locally advanced stages of the disease were incurable by radical surgery and often led to uncontrolled malignant ulceration across the chest wall. It is important to remember the clinical signs of breast cancer that would invalidate surgical attempts at cure, when initial referral to a medical oncologist would be more relevant (Table 3.2). Staging has also become important for selecting those patients who would most benefit from adjuvant systemic therapy (see Chapter 6), but these indices depend heavily on histological and biological variables. Thus anatomical mapping has become part of a broader staging strategy.

The staging systems currently in use are based on the clinical size and extent of invasion of the primary tumor (T), the clinical absence or

TABLE 3.2

Clinical signs precluding surgery

- Inflammatory changes throughout the breast
- Peau d'orange involving more than 30% of the surface area of the breast
- Ulceration of the skin (this is a relative contraindication; surgery may be technically possible for salvage)
- Fixation of the tumor to the underlying chest wall (fixation to the muscle alone is a relative contraindication that can be judged clinically; and surgery may be technically feasible for salvage)
- Fixation of the axillary lymph nodes to the chest wall or the neurovascular bundle supplying the arm
- Overt, distant metastatic disease, where the expectation of life is less than 2 years

presence of palpable axillary lymph nodes and evidence of their local invasion (N), together with the clinical and imaging evidence of distant metastases (M). This TNM classification (Table 3.3) has been subdivided into four broad categories by the Union Internationale Contre Cancer (UICC; Table 3.4). However, of these, only stage I localized to the breast and stage II with clinical lymph-node involvement of a limited extent are considered appropriate for primary treatment by surgery.

The principal measures used at present are invasion (a measure of invasive potential), nodal status (metastatic potential), tumor size (growth potential), histological grade (growth rate and regulatory potential) and hormone receptor status. In addition, a measure of overexpression of *HER2-neu*, an epithelial growth factor surface receptor, is now coming into use. Oddly, most staging systems do not take into account the growth rate of the primary tumor.

In addition to the classical clinical staging systems, more and more prognostic variables are being added, which may be mathematically subsumed into a global prognostic index. A well-known example of this is the Nottingham Prognostic Index (NPI; Table 3.5, page 44), which incorporates histological grade, tumor size and the extent of lymph-node infiltration.

TABLE 3.3

The tumor–nodes–metastases (TNM) classification of breast cancer

Tumor status

TX	Primary tumor cannot be assessed
T0	No evidence of primary tumor
Tis	Carcinoma in situ
T1	Tumor $\leq$ 2 cm
T1a	Tumor $\leq$ 0.5 cm
T1b	Tumor > 0.5 cm but < 1 cm
T1c	Tumor > 1 cm but < 2 cm
T2	Tumor > 2 cm but < 5 cm
T3	Tumor > 5 cm
T4	Tumor of any size with direct extension to the chest wall or skin
T4a	Extension to the chest wall
T4b	Edema (including peau d'orange), skin ulceration or satellite skin nodules confined to the same breast
T4c	Both T4a and T4b
T4d	Inflammatory carcinoma

Status of lymph nodes

NX	Regional lymph nodes cannot be assessed (e.g. removed previously)
N0	No regional lymph node metastasis
N1	Metastasis to movable ipsilateral axillary nodes
N2	Metastasis to ipsilateral axillary nodes with fixation
N3	Metastasis to ipsilateral internal mammary lymph nodes

Distant metastases

M0	No clinically apparent distant metastases
M1	Distant metastases obvious

Prognostic factors

It is reasonable to describe the natural history of breast cancer in terms of growth, invasion and metastatic potential. These properties are genetically controlled through the production of specific proteins.

TABLE 3.4

The Union Internationale Contre Cancer (UICC) staging system for breast cancer incorporating the TNM classification

UICC stage	TNM classification
I	T1, N0, M0
II	T1, N1, M0; T2, N0–1, M0*
III	Any T, N2–3, M0; T3, any N, M0; T4, any N, M0
IV	Any T, any N, M1

*Many expert groups include T2 tumors in stage I.

They are probably also time-dependent, with a tendency to become less controllable, and they are affected by the local milieu. Current prognostic indicators are largely indirect measures of these properties, and achieve about 60% accuracy.

Gene array technology offers the prospect of much greater precision. The system is based on the principle that each protein the body produces is the result of the activity of a particular gene (DNA), mediated through messenger RNA (mRNA). In a sense, array technology engineers the process in reverse.

The tissue sample is processed to extract mRNA, which is treated and exposed to a slide on which thousands of single-gene DNA fragments have been fixed in precisely identified positions. The processed mRNA (now cDNA) has a color tag, so that when it binds to complementary DNA on the slide, a tiny color spot can be seen (Figure 3.9). Comparisons can be made between tissues by tagging the cDNA from each tissue with a different color. If the colors are red and green, for example, and only one tissue expresses the gene, the dot will be red or green. If both tissues express the gene, the dot will be yellow. Thus tissues can be individually characterized and compared.

This approach is beginning to influence clinical medicine. Malignancies, particularly leukemias and lymphomas, are being classified by gene expression patterns in addition to conventional light microscopy and flow cytometry. Patterns of gene expression appear

TABLE 3.5

The Nottingham Prognostic Index

The figure shows prognostic sub-groups based on the Index

Histological grade	Score

To determine the grade, add the scores for each component:

3–5 = grade I; 6–7 = grade II; 8–9 = grade III

Tubule formation

Majority of tumor (> 75%)	1
Moderate amount (10–75%)	2
Little or none (< 10%)	3

Nuclear size

Regular, uniform	1
Larger variation	2
Marked variation	3

Mitotic frequency	Depends on microscope field size

Nodal stage

Node sampling: low axillary, apical axillary and internal mammary nodes

Stage A

Tumor absent from all nodes sampled at all three sites	1

Stage B

Tumor in a low axillary node only (or) in an internal mammary node only (or) in three or fewer nodes in an axillary clearance	2

Stage C

Tumor in apical node (or) in low axillary node plus internal mammary nodes (or) in four or more nodes in axillary clearance	3

Nottingham Prognostic Index = (0.2 x size in cm) + grade + stage

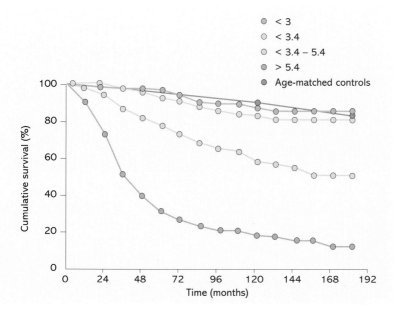

to correlate with light-microscopic diagnosis. Moreover, data are accumulating to allow clinicians to estimate the risk of relapse, its likely pattern and its response to specific treatments with greater precision. The current challenge is to make the technique sufficiently robust and reproducible for wider use.

Array technology has two promising practical advantages.

- It can be performed on very small samples, so needle and core biopsy at frequent intervals may allow more sophisticated monitoring.
- Variations of the technique can be used on archived samples, compressing the prognostication learning curve.

A further advantage is possible. As our understanding of breast cancer as a disease of regulation has become more refined, our treatments have become less anatomic: radical mastectomy has been replaced by less disfiguring surgeries; axillary node dissection is being superseded by sentinel node dissection. Perhaps gene array analysis of the primary tumor will provide sufficient information to obviate those procedures too. On the other hand, if the breast stem-cell hypothesis holds true, array technology may prove misleading, since the small number of critical stem cells will be lost in the mass of deranged tissue.

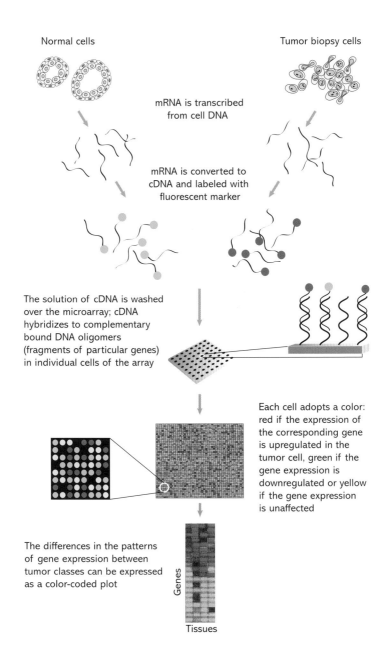

Normal cells

Tumor biopsy cells

mRNA is transcribed
from cell DNA

mRNA is converted to
cDNA and labeled with
fluorescent marker

The solution of cDNA is washed
over the microarray; cDNA
hybridizes to complementary
bound DNA oligomers
(fragments of particular genes)
in individual cells of the array

Each cell adopts a color:
red if the expression of
the corresponding gene
is upregulated in the
tumor cell, green if the
gene expression is
downregulated or yellow
if the gene expression
is unaffected

The differences in the patterns
of gene expression between
tumor classes can be expressed
as a color-coded plot

Genes

Tissues

Figure 3.9 Gene array technology.

Key points – pathophysiology

- Breast cancer is becoming understood as a constantly evolving series of defects in cellular regulation and control.
- Growth, invasion and metastasis are related but distinct regulatory processes. The mix determines the clinical course in an individual patient.
- Most breast lumps are benign, especially before age 50.
- Staging of breast cancer, including examination of lymph nodes, is a prognosis-estimating procedure. It is not therapeutic other than in achieving local control.
- New evidence is emerging that the act of surgery itself, or even major trauma at a later stage, might induce angiogenesis at the site of latent/occult distant metastases.
- Gene array techniques are bringing modern molecular biology into the clinic.

Key references

Dixon JM. Hormone replacement therapy and the breast. *BMJ* 2001;323:1381–2.

Hankinson SE, Willett WC, Colditz GA et al. Circulating concentrations of insulin-like growth factor-I and risk of breast cancer. *Lancet* 1998;351:1393–6.

Hedenfalk I, Duggan D, Chen Y et al. Gene expression profiles in hereditary breast cancer. *N Engl J Med* 2001;344:539.

Huang, E, Cheng SH, Dressman H et al. Gene expression predictors of breast cancer outcomes. *Lancet* 2003;361:1590–6.

Kelsey JL, Bernstein L. Epidemiology and prevention of breast cancer. *Annu Rev Public Health* 1996;17: 47–67.

Miller WR. *Estrogen and breast cancer*. Austin: RG Landes Company, 1996.

Ntzani EE, Ioannidis JPA. Predictive ability of DNA microarrays for cancer outcomes and correlates: an empirical assessment. *Lancet* 2003;362:1439–44.

Peto R, Boreham J, Clarke M et al. UK and USA breast cancer deaths down 25% in year 2000 at ages 29–60 years. *Lancet* 2000;355:1822.

Pike MC, Krailo MD, Henderson BE et al. 'Hormonal' risk factors, 'breast tissue age' and the age-incidence of breast cancer. *Nature* 1983; 303:767–70.

Santen RJ, Manni A, Harvey H et al. Endocrine treatment of breast cancer in women. *Endocr Rev* 1990;11: 221–65.

Thomas HV, Key TJ, Allen DS et al. A prospective study of endogenous serum hormone concentrations and breast cancer risk in post-menopausal women on the island of Guernsey. *Br J Cancer* 1997;76:401–5.

Symptoms of breast cancer

Although a lump in the breast is the most common presenting symptom of breast cancer, a variety of other symptoms may be present (Table 4.1).

Lumps resulting from breast cancer are generally single, hard and painless, and may be irregular in shape. Fibroadenomas, however, may also appear as single, hard lumps. Typically, breast cancers are about 2 cm in diameter by the time they become large enough to be palpable. Approximately 60% arise in the upper outer quadrant of the breast, but any area of the breast can be affected.

Pain in the breast is seldom due to cancer. The most common cause is the normal periodic pain during the menstrual cycle (cyclic mastalgia).

Bleeding from the nipple is a rare symptom of breast cancer; less than 3% of women report bleeding as a first symptom. The likelihood of

---

TABLE 4.1

Symptoms that may indicate breast cancer

- Lump in the breast
- Breast pain
- Changes in the size or shape of the breast
- Swelling of the arm (lymphedema)
- Dimpling of the skin of the breast
- Involution or inversion of the nipple
- Lump in the armpit
- Bleeding or discharge from the nipple
- Ulceration of the skin
- Symptoms of secondary tumors

cancer is increased if a lump is found on examination. In the absence of a lump, the most common cause of bleeding or bloodstained discharge is duct papilloma. Discharges from the nipple that are not bloodstained are usually due to duct ectasia in postmenopausal women. Discharges may also occur during early pregnancy, after breastfeeding, and during treatment with certain drugs, such as oral contraceptives, some antihypertensive agents and some antidepressants.

Changes in size or shape of the breasts may also indicate breast cancer. The affected breast may increase in size or become pendulous; conversely, in advanced breast cancer the breast may shrink owing to loss of normal breast tissue. The skin may dimple or pucker because of edema and infiltration of Cooper's ligaments, and the nipple may become inverted. The veins in the breast may become more prominent as the tumor enlarges.

Skin involvement. In advanced cases, the tumor may involve the skin, leading to ulceration (Figure 4.1). Blockage of the lymphatic circulation can cause lymphedema, resulting in swelling of the arm.

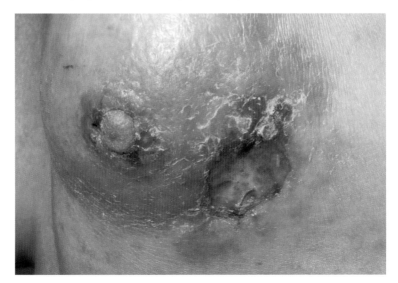

Figure 4.1 Ulcerating local recurrence in the breast and nipple after wide local excision and radiotherapy some years before.

Lymph nodes. Occasionally, it is not possible to identify the primary tumor, and the only evidence of breast cancer is enlarged lymph nodes.

Metastatic breast cancer can cause a variety of symptoms, including bone pain, breathlessness, nausea or jaundice.

When to refer?

Breast symptoms that require referral to a physician or clinic with a special interest in breast disease are summarized in Table 4.2. The following patient groups can be managed, at least initially, by the primary care physician:

- young women with tender, lumpy breasts and older women with symmetrical nodularity provided that no localized abnormality is present (Figure 4.2)
- women with minor or moderate breast pain who do not have a palpable lesion (Figure 4.3)
- women of any age who have nipple discharge that is from one or more ducts, or is intermittent, and is neither bloodstained nor troublesome (Figure 4.4).

There is no single test or group of tests that provides perfect accuracy in the diagnosis of breast cancer. An 'index of suspicion' remains the paramount principle. A suspect mass with negative mammographic findings warrants biopsy. Negative biopsy findings in such a patient should be reviewed for anatomical and histopathological accuracy.

Triple assessment

Triple assessment, which comprises clinical examination, imaging investigations and pathological evaluation, will enable a confident diagnosis in 95% of patients with suspected breast cancer (Figure 4.5).

Clinical examination is an essential first step in the diagnosis of breast cancer. The patient should be examined with her hands by her sides, above her head, and pressing on her hips. This can reveal nipple retraction, or asymmetry and dimpling of the breasts. The patient should then be asked to lie in a semirecumbent position and the breasts examined quadrant by quadrant with the flat of the hand (lubricating

TABLE 4.2

Symptoms requiring specialist referral

Lumps

- Any new discrete lump
- A new lump in pre-existing nodularity
- Asymmetrical nodularity persisting at review after menstruation
- Abscess
- Persistently refilling or recurrent cyst*
- Axillary or supraclavicular nodes

Pain

- Associated with a lump
- Intractable pain not responding to reassurance, simple measures such as wearing a well-fitting bra, or common drugs
- Persistent unilateral pain in postmenopausal women

Nipple discharge

- All women aged over 50 years
- Women aged below 50 years with:
  - bilateral discharge sufficient to stain clothes
  - bloodstained discharge
  - persistent discharge from a single duct

Nipple retraction or distortion, or nipple eczema

Change in skin contour

Family history

- A request from a woman with a strong family history of breast cancer (such patients should be referred to a family cancer genetics clinic where possible)

*Aspiration is acceptable if the patient has recurrent multiple cysts

the skin often makes this examination more sensitive). This procedure can distinguish between a distinct lump and coarse nodular tissue, which is a common feature of benign dysplasia. The axillary nodes and

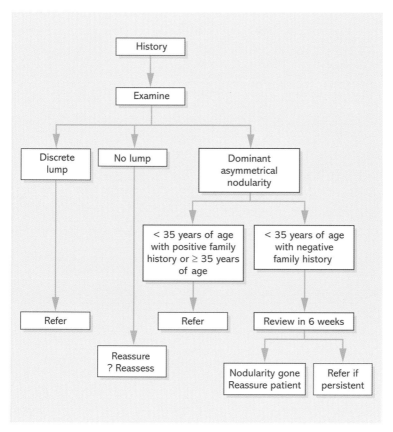

Figure 4.2 Guidelines for the management of patients with breast lumps.

supraclavicular nodes are then examined by palpation under the arms and above the collarbone.

Women who present with nipple discharge should be asked to massage the subareolar area to provoke secretion. The color and site of discharge should be noted; discharge from a single duct is usually due to a duct papilloma.

Imaging. Both mammography and ultrasonography have important roles in the diagnosis of breast cancer, but the use of other modalities, such as magnetic resonance and infrared imaging, is being developed.

Mammography has a diagnostic accuracy of over 95% for clinically detectable tumors, and approximately 50% for subclinical cancers.

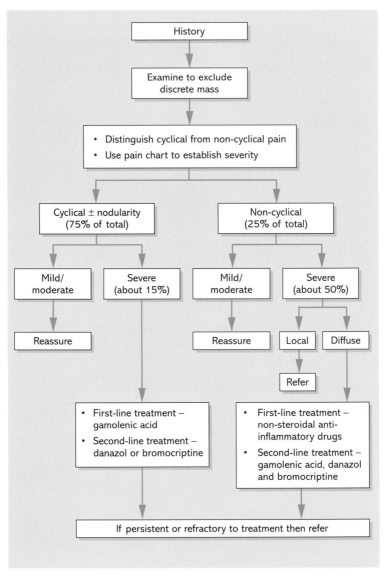

Figure 4.3 Guidelines for the management of patients with breast pain.

The technique can provide single oblique views of each breast, or both lateral and craniocaudal views. However, because it involves compressing the breast between two plates, the procedure can be uncomfortable.

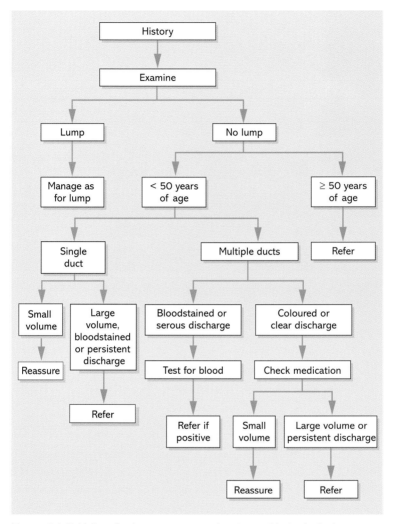

Figure 4.4 Guidelines for the management of patients with nipple discharge.

Although mammography contributes little to the management of a patient with a discrete, palpable lump, in whom the diagnosis should be based on cytology and histology if appropriate, it does have an important role in specific situations.

- Mammography may increase the likelihood of detecting a relatively small cancer in patients whose breasts have a coarse, nodular texture.

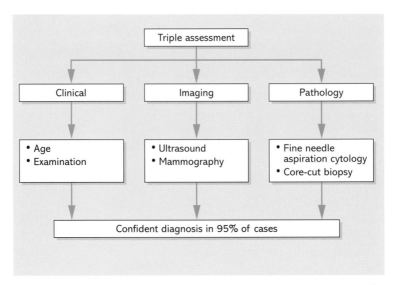

Figure 4.5 Triple assessment enables a confident diagnosis to be made in 95% of patients with suspected breast cancer.

- The technique can be used to locate the cancer accurately for excision biopsy (Figure 4.6).
- In women with a palpable lump, mammography may reveal an impalpable lump in the same or opposite breast. Mammography should therefore be a prerequisite before conservative breast surgery is undertaken.
- Women who have undergone mastectomy for breast cancer are at increased risk of developing cancer in the remaining breast, and thus regular mammography may be useful for monitoring the contralateral breast.

Mammography is also mandatory for localizing impalpable tumors prior to surgery (Figure 4.6).

Ultrasonography is becoming more widely used in the evaluation of clinical abnormalities in the breast.

- Ultrasound has a specificity of nearly 100% in distinguishing a solid mass from a cystic mass (Figure 4.7); the diagnosis can then be confirmed and treated by simple needle aspiration. Improvements in technology have also increased both the sensitivity and specificity of ultrasound in the diagnosis of solid breast lumps. Benign lumps

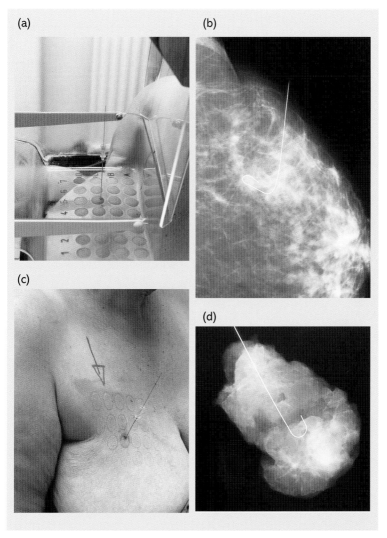

Figure 4.6 Mammography can be used to locate the tumor accurately before open biopsy. (a) Under local anesthesia, the breast is compressed in the mammogram unit and a needle inserted through a grid overlying the suspected tumor location. (b) Craniocaudal and oblique mammograms are then taken to ensure that the needle is lying close to the tumor. (c) The patient is next taken to the operating theater with the needle in situ. (d) The needle and the suspected tumor are excised and sent for radiological examination to confirm that the suspect area has been removed before the wound is closed.

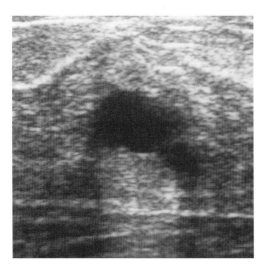

Figure 4.7 Simple cyst shown on ultrasound scan. Note the smooth margins, hypoechoic center and posterior acoustic enhancement.

are well circumscribed with no acoustic shadow or isodense echoes, whereas malignant lumps have irregular outlines, are poorly defined and are variable in density or have echoes suggestive of microcalcifications.

- Distinguishing discrete lumps from areas of nodularity in a relatively young woman can be difficult. Ultrasound can provide reassurance if it fails to detect any localized abnormality.

- Ultrasound is used routinely to guide fine-needle aspiration cytology and to localize subclinical lesions with needles prior to excision biopsy.

- Although it has not yet replaced axillary node dissection, the use of ultrasound with enhanced color Doppler assessment of blood flow is, at present, one of the most promising approaches to the preoperative assessment of axillary metastases. In addition to detecting masses, it can detect increased vascularity, which can indicate lymph-node involvement.

- Enhanced color Doppler ultrasound scanning of the breast postoperatively is likely to improve the early diagnosis of local recurrence, which is otherwise difficult to achieve because of surgical scarring and the effects of radiotherapy.

Magnetic resonance. In the past few years, there has been an explosion of interest in magnetic resonance imaging (MRI) of the breast. This technique, which is based on the nuclear spin of molecules within a powerful magnetic field, is free of the hazards of conventional X-ray imaging. It produces remarkable digitized images that allow three-dimensional reconstruction of the breast (Figure 4.8a). Furthermore, injection of a contrast agent enables the vascularity of the lesion of interest to be visualized either as a dynamic function of uptake or as a static image (Figure 4.8b). However, the images are expensive to acquire and need an experienced team of radiologist and surgeon to utilize them appropriately.

The technology is exciting and, in certain circumstances, may aid in the diagnosis and management of the disease. However, in the authors' opinion, the precise role of MRI awaits formal assessment. In addition, caution should be exercised to avoid the over-representation of 'latent' lesions at a distance from the dominant primary, which may persuade some surgeons to ignore the clinical trials of the past by offering mastectomy, when all the evidence would point to the safety of breast-conserving techniques.

Pathology. If a discrete lump is present, a test aspiration can be performed with a 20-mL syringe and venipuncture needle. If the lump is due to a cyst, aspiration will provide immediate relief and reassurance. A bloodstained aspirate may indicate the presence of an intracystic cancer requiring open biopsy (see page 61). If the lump is solid, fine-needle aspiration can be used to obtain cells for cytological examination which, in some centers, can be completed within 30 minutes. Ideally, an

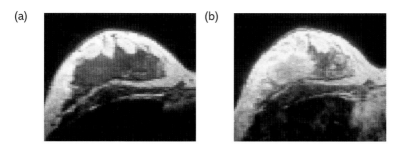

(a) (b)

Figure 4.8 Typical MRI appearance of breast cancer (a) before and (b) after the injection of an enhancing agent. Reproduced courtesy of Mr Michael Douek.

ultrasound scan should be performed before needle aspiration, as this will accurately predict whether the lump is solid or cystic.

Fine-needle aspiration cytology (FNAC) was popularized in Sweden decades ago and has been widely adopted in the rest of Europe in recent years, but is still less used in the USA. The technique is simple, and a skilled operator can usually produce an adequate sample from very small tumors by inserting the needle either into a clinically palpable lump or stereotactically under radiological or ultrasound control. The aspirate is immediately smeared on a series of slides and stained for conventional microscopic examination (Figure 4.9).

Experienced cytopathologists can diagnose breast cancer with almost 100% specificity. The sensitivity (i.e. false-negative rate) depends to a large extent on the operating skills of the clinician taking the sample and the experience of the cytologist. In many centers around the world where cytopathology results have been audited, surgeons are happy to carry out definitive cancer surgery on this result alone.

Biopsy. If cytological examination of cells obtained by FNAC is equivocal, a core biopsy can be obtained using a cutting needle technique under local anesthesia. Histological examination of the sample can then be used to confirm the diagnosis of cancer; open biopsy should be performed if a negative result is obtained, to exclude the possibility of cancer cells being present elsewhere in the lump. Nevertheless, modern core-cut biopsy techniques are considered the 'standard of care', particularly for lesions detected on screening.

(a) (b)

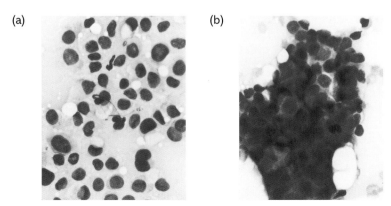

Figure 4.9 Examples of (a) malignant and (b) benign cytology.

Open biopsy involves the removal of the entire lump under general anesthesia. This procedure is associated with considerable morbidity; approximately 20% of patients develop a further lump under the scar, or experience pain at the biopsy site. Thus, it should only be performed in patients who have been fully investigated by fine-needle aspiration cytology, mammography and core biopsy, and in whom the diagnosis still remains equivocal (Table 4.3).

Breast screening and breast awareness

The aim of screening for breast cancer is to reduce mortality by detecting tumors before they have spread beyond the breast. Similarly, since over 90% of breast cancers are first detected by the woman herself, the rationale for regular self-examination is to increase the likelihood of detecting a tumor at the smallest size possible.

Screening. There is evidence that screening for breast cancer by regular mammography can reduce mortality from breast cancer by 20–30% in certain groups when compared with that in unscreened women of the same age. Significant benefits, however, are seen only in women over the age of 50 years. In trials in Sweden, for example, mortality during 12 years of follow-up was reduced by 29% in women over 50 years of age, compared with only 13% in younger women. Furthermore, the reduction in younger women was not statistically significant, and was delayed by at least 8 years. There is, therefore, no evidence to support regular screening in women less than 50 years of age. This is an ongoing controversy.

TABLE 4.3

Indications for open biopsy

- Cytological diagnosis of malignancy that is not supported by results of other investigations
- Suspicion of malignancy on one or more investigations, even when other investigations suggest that the lesion is probably benign

It is worth noting that consumer advocacy groups also hold this viewpoint. The National Breast Cancer Coalition (NBCC) in the USA states: 'Women deserve to know the truth – and the truth is that there is no evidence of a mortality reduction in women under the age of 50 and the evidence for women over the age of 50 is currently unclear. Broad public health recommendations should only be made when it is clear that the potential benefits of the recommended intervention will outweigh the potential harms. NBCC believes that women are capable of educating themselves so that they can make their own individual decisions about screening.'

Screening programs for breast cancer are associated with a number of problems (see also Box 11.3, page 140).

- Only about 70% of women accept mammography, and there is some evidence that these women have a higher incidence of breast problems than expected.
- It is possible that a woman who is reassured by a negative result might ignore changes in her breasts between mammograms. Since approximately 20–30% of breast cancers are not detected by mammography, some tumors could, therefore, be missed.
- False-positive results are obtained in about 1% of mammograms. Such results could generate unnecessary anxiety, particularly if further investigations are undertaken.
- For every breast cancer detected, a substantial number of women will undergo biopsies or surgery for benign breast disease, with attendant morbidity.
- Although the total dose of radiation received during mammography is low (< 1.5 mGy), it has been suggested that repeated exposure could increase the risk of breast cancer. This risk is, however, low. It has been estimated that screening 2 million women over 50 years of age by a single mammogram would result in one extra case of breast cancer each year after 10 years; by contrast, the normal incidence of breast cancer in women over 60 years of age is approximately 2000 cases/million.
- Small breast cancers detected by mammography may be biologically different from those detected clinically. Approximately 20% of cancers detected by mammography are carcinomas in situ, some of

which would never progress to invasive disease if left undetected, and the optimal treatment for such tumors is unknown. If these cancers are treated in the same way as invasive cancers, some women may undergo unnecessarily extensive surgery. Conversely, in other women, delaying treatment of asymptomatic disease may ultimately compromise the chance of cure.

• The optimum interval between mammograms has not been determined. The UK screening program currently recommends screening at 3-year intervals, but this is judged to be too long by some advocates of screening. Yet to shorten the interval would have major cost implications. Thus, although radiographic screening is 'standard of care' in many places, it remains controversial.

Breast self-examination. Several large-scale programs have been established to teach self-examination techniques and encourage women to examine their breasts each month. However, although this approach does appear to lead to the detection of smaller tumors, there is no evidence that it improves long-term survival. Indeed, in a recent large-scale, randomized, controlled trial performed in St Petersburg (formerly Leningrad), there was no difference in breast cancer mortality rates between people trained in breast self-examination and a control group. An adverse effect of the training in self-examination was the disproportionate number of women presenting with lumpy breasts who were then subjected to futile biopsies. There is also a potential problem with the self-examination approach in that random biopsies among premenopausal women may disclose ductal carcinoma in situ or lobular carcinoma in situ, whose natural history is unknown. Such findings may result in inappropriate radical surgery or, at the very least, a lifetime of uncertainty and anxiety for the patient.

In July 2001, the Canadian Medical Association went one step further when it published new guidelines following a systematic review of the literature. As a public health measure, self-examination was relegated from category C (of no proven value) to category D (of proven harm)! This report, as expected, provoked storms of protest on both sides of the Atlantic. The controversy has deep roots. Part of the difficulty lies in the intuitive notion that detecting a tumor 'earlier'

TABLE 4.4

'Breast awareness' – changes for which medical advice should be sought

- Dimpling or flaking of the skin
- Nipple discharge
- New lump or thickening in the breast tissue, particularly if not cyclic
- Unusual pain or discomfort
- Any *new* difference in the appearance of the breasts (when looking at them, lifting them, or moving the arms)

(i.e. when it is smaller) is necessarily better, but it is becoming apparent that not all breast cancers are the same, even if they appear so morphologically. Thus the disappointing results with early diagnostic attempts, including both imaging and self-examination, probably reflect our incomplete understanding of breast cancer as a process.

In the UK, emphasis has recently switched to 'breast awareness' rather than regular self-examination. In this approach, women are encouraged to become familiar with their breasts and to distinguish between normal cyclic fluctuations and abnormal changes for which medical advice should be sought (Table 4.4). This can be done by feeling the breasts with a soapy hand while washing. The breast awareness approach should allow prompt reassurance to be given in most cases, and increase the likelihood that conservative surgery would be possible if breast cancer were detected.

Key points – diagnosis

- A logical process for assessing breast pain or masses will greatly enhance diagnostic accuracy.
- Clinical examination plus imaging plus pathological examination (triple assessment) represent the diagnostic gold standard.
- No test is pathognomonic. Clinical judgment has high value.
- In coming years, staging will rely less on anatomic/morphological observations and will be based more on regulatory process and 'molecular' grounds using gene array techniques.
- Breast screening programs have modest utility. Their greatest value may be in increasing patient self-awareness and in the improved organization of clinical services.
- Breast self-examination can no longer be recommended, although women should be aware of normal physiological changes and thus be alerted to the first chance observation of a pathological change.

Key references

Baxter N, Canadian Task Force on Preventive Health Care. Preventive health care, 2001 update: should women be routinely taught breast self-examination to screen for breast cancer? *CMAJ* 2001;164;1837–46.

Mettlin CJ, Smart CR. The Canadian National Breast Screening Study. An appraisal and implications for early detection policy. *Cancer* 1993;72: 1461–5.

Nekhlyudov L, Fletcher SW. Is it time to stop teaching breast self-examination? *CMAJ* 2001;164:1851.

Nystrom L, Andersson I, Bjurstam N et al. Long-term effects of mammography screening: updated overview of the Swedish randomized trials. *Lancet* 2002;359:909–19.

Tabar L, Fagerberg G, Duffy SW et al. The Swedish two county trial of mammographic screening for breast cancer: recent results and calculation of benefit. *J Epidemiol Community Health* 1989;43:107–14.

Walloch J. Technique and interpretation of breast aspiration cytology. *Clin Obstet Gynecol* 1989;32:786–99.

It is now recognized that breast cancer is a systemic disease at the time of clinical diagnosis in most cases. The disease originates in the breast, but has more widespread manifestations. The malignant potential of an individual cancer manifests early, and most breast cancers that have the potential to metastasize do so before clinical diagnosis is possible. Long-term follow-up studies have clearly shown that the risks of recurrence and death correlate with disease stage at diagnosis. Thus, the goal of staging is to gather adequate prognostic information to guide therapy, taking into account the associated risks. It is important to establish:
- the origin and type of the tumor
- how far the tumor has spread
- other factors, such as menopausal status and the presence of concomitant disease, that may influence the treatment plan.
  The goals of treatment are:
- to prevent or delay recurrence for as long as possible where there is no evident disease
- to relieve symptoms and improve quality of life in patients in whom distant metastases are present at diagnosis (this group accounts for about 10% of new diagnoses in most Western countries).

Since breast cancer is a systemic disease, therapies such as radiotherapy and surgery are used to achieve local control, and systemic treatments (chemotherapy, immunotherapy, hormonal treatment) are used to alter the systemic milieu and attack distant metastases. However, recent evidence suggests that inadequate local control is associated with an increase of nearly 5% in breast-cancer-specific deaths. Local and systemic therapies are not necessarily used sequentially, but are mixed to maximize benefit and minimize risk according to the needs of the individual patient.

Treatment of primary cancer

Beyond removal of the primary tumor, local treatments such as surgery or radiation have only a modest effect on overall survival. These treatments are used mainly for diagnostic purposes and to reduce the likelihood of local recurrence within the breast, chest wall or axillary nodes. Systemic therapies, including chemotherapy and hormonal manipulation, reduce the risk of both local and systemic recurrence and, to some extent, improve survival. While primary breast surgery has long been the first step in treatment, there is no evidence that this policy should be rigidly adhered to. Indeed, where local control is unlikely to be achieved, for example in inflammatory carcinomas and extensive local disease, primary surgery may be contraindicated; distant metastases are another relative contraindication. The main indication for primary surgery is the realistic opportunity to achieve long-term disease-free survival or effective cure.

It is not surprising, given our appreciation that breast cancer is a systemic disease, that even in early, localized breast cancer, the sequence of treatments is being reconsidered. Trials of systemic treatment before definitive surgery are being undertaken in an approach that has been termed 'neoadjuvant' therapy. After a confirmatory biopsy and baseline imaging, a course of chemotherapy and/or hormone manipulation is given. The primary tumor is then assessed for a response, and surgery with possible additional radiation treatment follows. In some trials, the observed response to chemotherapy appears to be a predictor of long-term, disease-free survival. Most randomized, controlled clinical trials so far have reported that the possibility of carrying out breast-conserving surgery is increased by neoadjuvant therapy. However, the impact of this resequencing on survival is not yet known.

Surgical treatment of primary cancer

The aims of surgical treatment for primary breast cancer are to:
- achieve cure in patients in whom the disease is confined to the breast
- achieve local control of the disease, to prevent complications such as skin ulceration
- determine the pathological stage of lymph-node involvement
- obtain sufficient tumor for measurement of estrogen receptor status and other prognostic markers.

Surgery may consist of either mastectomy or conservative procedures, so-called 'lumpectomies' (Table 5.1).

TABLE 5.1

Surgical options in breast cancer

Procedure	Advantages	Disadvantages
Conservative surgery	• Breast retained • No need for prosthesis	• Postoperative radiotherapy indicated • Risk of local recurrence requiring delayed surgery of 1%/year • Difficulty in monitoring • Cosmetic results often disappointing
Total (simple) mastectomy	• Postoperative radiotherapy not usually required • Avoids the surgical morbidity associated with dissection of the axilla	• Radiotherapy may be required to control axillary disease • Little information about staging available from the lymph nodes to guide systemic therapy • External prosthesis or major surgery for reconstruction required
Modified (Patey) radical mastectomy	• Postoperative radiotherapy, including to the axilla, not usually required • Staging information from the lymph nodes available	• External prosthesis or radical mastectomy major surgery for reconstruction required
Classical (Halsted) radical mastectomy (rarely done)	• May help to achieve local control of indolent, advanced disease that has failed to respond to radiotherapy or systemic therapy	• Ugly appearance that is difficult to mask with a prosthesis • Breast reconstruction difficult

Mastectomy. The most commonly used mastectomy procedures are the simple (or total) mastectomy and the modified radical (Patey's) mastectomy.

Simple mastectomy. The entire breast tissue, including the axillary tail, is removed together with the skin, nipple and areola (Figure 5.1). Samples from the lowest axillary lymph nodes are usually also taken.

Modified radical mastectomy removes the same structures as simple mastectomy, together with the pectoralis minor muscle. This allows easy removal of the axillary lymph nodes, without greatly increasing the amount of tissue removed. In both cases, the use of a prosthesis (see pages 75 and 117) allows women to wear swimming costumes or low necklines.

Subcutaneous mastectomy. In a small number of women, it is possible to remove most of the breast tissue while leaving the skin and nipple intact. The breast can then be reconstructed immediately with an implant. This procedure is, however, mainly used in women with high-risk precancerous conditions such as carcinoma in situ.

Complications. The most common complications after mastectomy are wound infections and shoulder weakness (Table 5.2). Lymphedema

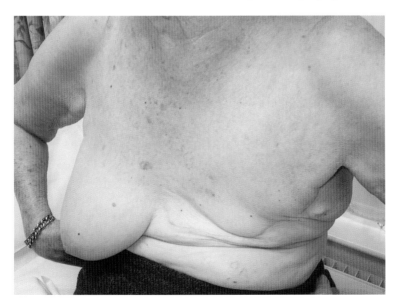

Figure 5.1 The typical appearance of mastectomy in an elderly woman.

TABLE 5.2

Complications after mastectomy for primary breast cancer

- Wound complications
  - bruising
  - swelling
  - delayed healing
  - infection
  - damaged intercostal brachial nerve
- Shoulder weakness or stiffness
- Swelling of arm due to lymphedema

resulting from damage to the lymph nodes is becoming rarer as radical procedures are performed less frequently. Shoulder movement can be restored by postoperative physiotherapy (see Chapter 8).

Conservative procedures include:
- wide local excision, in which the lump is removed with a 1-cm margin of normal tissue
- quadrantectomy, in which an entire quadrant is removed (Figure 5.2).

With adjuvant radiotherapy, these procedures produce comparable survival to that achieved with mastectomy (Figure 5.3). However, conservative surgery is not suitable for all patients; the outcome is influenced by a number of factors, including the size of the tumor relative to the size of the breast, and the stage and grade of the tumor (Table 5.3). Moreover, many women opt for mastectomy because of a need to feel that the tumor has been completely eradicated, or because of an unwillingness to accept adjuvant radiotherapy. Thus, the choice of operation should be discussed with the patient and her family.

Treatment of regional lymph nodes

The indications for axillary surgery and the extent to which it should be carried out in women with operable breast cancer remain controversial. This is mainly the result of confusion regarding the changing role of

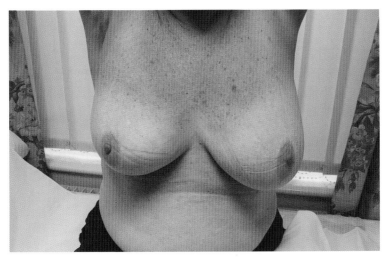

Figure 5.2 The typical appearance after breast-conserving surgery.

axillary dissection over the last two decades. Initially, it was thought that axillary surgery in its own right might improve survival, but this belief is no longer tenable. There is also concern that, without surgery, uncontrolled axillary disease, which can lead to lymphedema and paralysis of the arm, would occur in a significant number of women. In terms of local control, however, there may be little to choose between the success of surgery and the success of radiotherapy, balanced against the relatively rare, but significant, morbidity of either approach. It is, however, likely that axillary surgery will have a decreasing role in the future, partly because of the earlier presentation of the disease and partly because of improvements in the prognostic value of tumor markers.

TABLE 5.3

Breast cancers suitable for conservative surgery

- Single clinical and mammographic lesion
- Tumor ≤ 4 cm
- No local advancement (T1, T2 < 4 cm), extensive nodal involvement (N0, N1), or metastases (M0)
- Tumor > 4 cm in a large breast

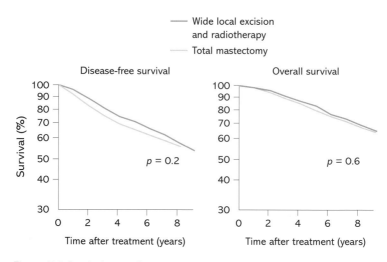

Figure 5.3 Survival rates after conservative surgery for primary breast cancer are comparable to those after mastectomy. The figure shows disease-free and overall survival in patients treated by mastectomy or by wide local excision followed by radiotherapy.

Axillary surgery. If axillary dissection is necessary, the technique used must reduce the morbidity of the procedure as much as possible. One of the most common postoperative problems is anesthesia or paresthesia in the axilla and the medial aspect of the arm, which results from surgical division of the intercostal brachial nerve. In skilled hands, this complication is easily avoided by identifying the nerve as it emerges from the medial aspect of the axilla through an intercostal space, and dissecting it all the way down to re-entry in the upper arm. Restriction of shoulder movements can be avoided by physiotherapy, and is less of a problem if the pectoralis minor is not divided.

Lymphedema of the arm is now relatively uncommon provided that the surgical clearance of the axilla is limited to the inferior surface of the axillary vein and the medial border of pectoralis minor. Radiotherapy should not be given after axillary surgery unless there is evidence of extranodal spread of the disease.

Prognosis. The most contentious area remains the role of the axillary dissection to establish the prognosis and thereby to help select appropriate systemic therapy. In such cases, surgery is only warranted if knowledge of the lymph-node status would change the approach to therapy. For example, at one extreme, a 30-year-old woman with a grade III primary cancer would almost certainly be expected to receive adjuvant systemic chemotherapy, irrespective of the lymph-node status. At the other extreme, in a woman over the age of 60 years with a small well-differentiated cancer and a low probability of lymph-node involvement, adjuvant systemic chemotherapy would not be used even in the presence of positive lymph nodes if local policy was to prescribe tamoxifen. In between these extremes, there are many cases where knowledge of the lymph-node status might influence the decision to prescribe chemotherapy. Having decided to embark on axillary surgery, most surgeons would accept a level II or III dissection to achieve both local control and staging; a level I dissection might be considered too much of a compromise. However, this procedure is not particularly therapeutic and carries considerable morbidity – thus the desire for a more selective diagnostic procedure.

Sentinel node biopsy. A more recent and potentially exciting development, which may avoid the need for a large number of negative axillary dissections, is sentinel node biopsy; indeed this technique is rapidly becoming the 'standard of care' in many parts of the world.

It is now recognized that most breast cancers spread in a predictable path along the axillary lymphatics with the lowermost node in the chain (the sentinel node) being the first to be affected. The biological basis of this procedure is that examining the axillary nodes provides prognostic information about the risk of systemic recurrence. A negative sentinel node with skip lesions higher up the axilla occurs in only about 3% of cases.

The sentinel node can be identified either by using an injection of a vital dye or by injecting a radioactive isotope bound to colloidal albumin, with a hand-held γ-counter to guide the surgeon to the appropriate lymph node. This procedure can be carried out before the definitive operation, or by using frozen section at time of surgery. If the sentinel node is negative, it is reasonable not to explore the axilla any further and, if positive, to proceed to a formal axillary dissection; a large series justifying this approach has been reported by Veronesi et al. It is possible, if not probable, that in coming years equal or better prognostic information will be gained from the primary tumor.

ALMANAC (axillary lymph-node mapping axillary node clearance) is a randomized, UK trial to compare sentinel node biopsy and conventional axillary node dissection, and is now close to completion.

In this study, surgeons have a learning phase of 40 cases in which they have to demonstrate that they can identify the sentinel node with a success rate of over 90%. Thereafter, they can join a multicenter trial in which patients are randomized to management according to the result of the sentinel node biopsy or to conventional axillary node dissection. Outcome measures include patient satisfaction, short-term morbidity, locoregional relapse and survival. The results of this study presented so far have demonstrated a significant reduction in morbidity, and an improvement in quality of life and patient satisfaction, after sentinel node biopsy.

Studies of similar design are in progress in the USA and Italy. As in the UK, expertise and experience in the sentinel node procedure are implicit requirements. Major institutions have tended to require surgeons to have performed sentinel node biopsy followed by axillary dissection in a substantial number of patients in order to achieve an acceptable standard of expertise.

Reconstructive surgery

Breast reconstruction following mastectomy is becoming increasingly popular, though currently only about 5% of patients undergo such surgery. The aims of reconstructive surgery are to:
- restore the natural breast contour as far as possible
- establish symmetry between the new mound and the remaining breast
- to produce a pleasing nipple–areola complex.

Ideally, breast reconstruction should be performed at the same time as the initial mastectomy as this reduces the psychological impact of losing a breast and avoids the need for further surgery. In practice, however, this may not be feasible, as both a cancer surgeon and a plastic surgeon are needed. A number of options for breast reconstruction are available (Table 5.4).

TABLE 5.4

Options for breast reconstruction

- Silicone gel implants
- Tissue expanders and prostheses
- Myocutaneous flaps
  - latissimus dorsi
  - transverse rectus abdominis

Silicone gel implants offer the simplest approach to reconstruction, and are suitable for women with small breasts. The implant is placed high on the chest wall, beneath the pectoralis major muscle. The full effect is not achieved until several months after surgery, when the skin and surrounding tissues have stretched to accommodate the implant. Careful adjustment of the size and position of the remaining breast is necessary to achieve a symmetrical appearance. There is no scientific evidence that silicone implants are associated with any health hazard, including autoimmune disease.

Tissue expanders. This approach involves implanting an inflatable bag which is filled with saline via a subcutaneous valve implanted in the patient's side. About 50 mL of saline is injected at 1–2 week intervals, until the breast mound is about 1.5 times larger than the remaining breast (so that the breast will hang naturally when the bag is removed). The bag is then removed and replaced with a silicone implant at a second operation. Recent devices such as the Becker prosthesis incorporate a silicone prosthesis (Figure 5.4) and so only the valve needs to be removed, which can be done under local anesthetic.

Myocutaneous flaps. This technique involves using a flap of skin and muscle to recreate the breast mound. This approach is useful in women with large breasts, or in whom a large amount of tissue was removed, or in cases where the skin is unlikely to accommodate an implant (e.g. after radiotherapy). The two most common reconstructions involve the rectus abdominis (transverse rectus abdominis myocutaneous [TRAM] flap) or latissimus dorsi muscles (Figure 5.5).

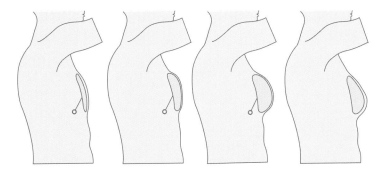

Figure 5.4 In the Becker breast reconstruction technique, a silicone prosthesis containing a tissue expander filled via a subcutaneous valve is used to create a new breast mound. The valve is subsequently removed under local anesthetic.

If desired, the nipple can be reconstructed surgically to give a reasonable cosmetic appearance. Tissue can be taken from the other nipple or, if necessary, from the thigh or labia. This operation should be performed several months after mastectomy to allow the reconstructed breast to attain its final shape, so that the heights of the nipples can be matched.

Radiotherapy

Radiotherapy is mandatory for most patients undergoing conservative surgery, and is considered appropriate for women at high risk of recurrence after mastectomy, such as:

- women with a large primary tumor, particularly if the tumor is poorly differentiated
- women with lymph-node involvement who have not undergone full axillary clearance
- women with involvement of the pectoralis major muscle.

Treatment is normally given in 3–5-weekly sessions for up to 6 weeks. The most common side effects are skin reactions and, occasionally, nausea and vomiting; pneumonitis resulting from irradiation of the lung occurs in fewer than 2% of patients.

Meta-analysis data released in late 2004, covering 79 trials (about 42 000 women over as long as 20 years), yield the following conclusions.

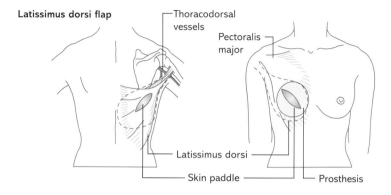

Latissimus dorsi flap

Thoracodorsal vessels

Pectoralis major

Latissimus dorsi

Skin paddle

Prosthesis

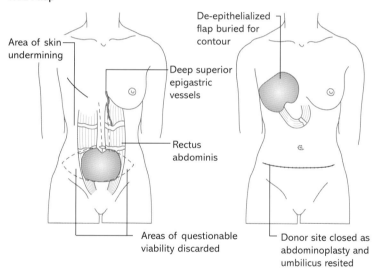

TRAM flap

Area of skin undermining

De-epithelialized flap buried for contour

Deep superior epigastric vessels

Rectus abdominis

Areas of questionable viability discarded

Donor site closed as abdominoplasty and umbilicus resited

Figure 5.5 Breast reconstruction by myocutaneous flap can involve either latissimus dorsi or transverse rectus abdominis myocutaneous (TRAM) flaps.

- Radiotherapy provides highly effective local control, preventing local recurrence in more than 80% of those treated (Figure 5.6).
- A small but statistically highly significant increase in death rate of about 4% is observed after 15 years, subsequent to local recurrence.
- Cardiac side effects for local tumors are significant, but the trend is to fewer complications with modern treatment approaches.

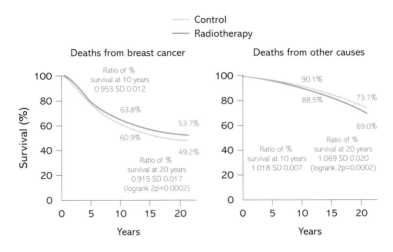

Figure 5.6 Radiotherapy reduces the incidence of local recurrence after mastectomy, but does not affect overall survival.

Furthermore, it would appear that if radiation damage to the left anterior descending coronary artery can be avoided, then similar gains in survival are achievable in high-risk patients undergoing mastectomy.

Intraoperative radiotherapy following local excision of early breast cancer is a recently developed technique that is currently under study. One such system, the Intrabeam (Figure 5.7), which was developed at University College, London, UK, is a completely portable unit that can be utilized in any operating theater without special shielding to deliver targeted radiotherapy. It is of great potential value in the management of early breast cancer treated by breast-conserving techniques. Modern understanding of breast cancer pathology now suggests that occult/ latent lesions in areas of the breast remote from the index quadrant are not the reason for local relapse, which almost always occurs at the site of the original excision. (Indeed, as Veronesi has pointed out, a cancer is just as likely to develop in the contralateral breast as a recurrence outside the index quadrant in the ipsilateral breast, yet we would never consider prophylactic radiotherapy to the other side!) If that is indeed the case, then carefully targeted high-dose radiotherapy at the time of surgery may obviate the need for external beam therapy, thus saving

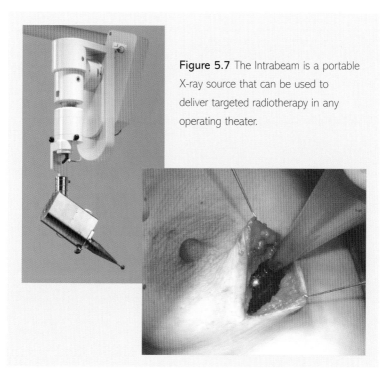

Figure 5.7 The Intrabeam is a portable X-ray source that can be used to deliver targeted radiotherapy in any operating theater.

machine time and the patient's time, in addition to opening up the possibility of breast conservation for breast cancer among women in the developing world; in most developing countries and many parts of the developed world, journeys are so long and/or tiring as to make breast-conserving surgery a non-viable option. Furthermore, by

Key points – local control of primary tumor

- Mastectomy and lumpectomy plus radiation are therapeutically equivalent for most women.
- Given adequate information, women choose equally between mastectomy and breast conservation approaches.
- Breast reconstruction is a viable alternative.
- In the future, selected patients may be able to avoid 6 weeks of conventional postoperative radiotherapy with a single dose of partial breast radiotherapy in the intra- or perioperative period.

applying the walls of the excision cavity to the applicator after tumorectomy, the conformal geometry is much better than the simulations required for external beam treatment, which should in theory lead to better local control of the disease.

Other techniques with a similar rationale include 'ELLIOT', which was developed in the European breast cancer center in Milan, and the mammosite technique. Although they are attractive, the outcome of randomized controlled trials must be awaited to define the appropriate clinical settings for their use.

Key references

Breast Surgeons Group of the British Association of Surgical Oncology. Guidelines for surgeons in the management of symptomatic breast disease in the United Kingdom. *Eur J Surg Oncol* 1995;21:1–13.

Early Breast Cancer Trialists' Collaborative Group. Systemic treatment of early breast cancer by hormonal, cytotoxic, or immune therapy; 133 randomised trials involving 31 000 recurrences and 24 000 deaths among 75 000 women. *Lancet* 1992;339:1–5.

Goldhirsch A, Wood WC, Senn H-J et al. Meeting highlights: International Consensus Panel on the Treatment of Primary Breast Cancer. *J Natl Cancer Inst* 1995;87:1441–5.

Houghton J, Baum M, Haybittle JL. Role of radiotherapy following total mastectomy in patients with early breast cancer. The Closed Trials Working Party of the CRC Breast Cancer Trials Group. *World J Surg* 1994;18:117–22.

Sacks NP, Baum M. Primary management of carcinoma of the breast. *Lancet* 1993;342:1402–8.

Sainsbury R, Haward B, Rider L et al. Influence of clinician workload and patterns of treatment on survival from breast cancer. *Lancet* 1995; 345:1265–70.

Vaidya JS, Tobias JS, Baum M et al. Intraoperative radiotherapy for breast cancer. *Lancet Oncol* 2004; 5:165–73.

Veronesi U, Paganelli G, Galimberti V et al. Sentinel-node biopsy to avoid axillary node dissection in breast cancer with clinically negative lymph nodes. *Lancet* 1997;349:1864–7.

While surgery and radiation offer local control of the primary tumor, systemic therapies aim to prevent or delay distant metastases. This is called 'adjuvant' therapy and marks the most significant change in breast cancer management in the past 25 years. Data have shown unequivocally that adjuvant therapy provides significant and prolonged improvement in survival. Indeed, the approximately 30% fall in breast cancer mortality in the UK since 1985, from an all-time high in the late 1970s, has mainly been ascribed to the widespread adoption of adjuvant systemic therapy. Similar data have been obtained in North America.

Adjuvant therapy is based on two principles. First, at least in animal models, there is a burst of mitotic activity in metastatic sites after a primary tumor is removed. This has been attributed variably to removal of growth inhibitory factors released by the primary tumor, surgical suppression of 'immunity' or activation of angiogenesis. Secondly, breast cancer is a systemic disease characterized by widespread early occult metastasis, which usually antedates diagnosis. Thus the clinical evolution of a particular breast cancer is a function of the activity of these remote and very occult micrometastases. Careful examination of survival curves stratified by stage at diagnosis shows that the hazard ratio, or the proportionate likelihood of recurrence, increases with stage classification. This suggests that tumors at different anatomic stages are some how biologically different, providing another element in the rationale for adjuvant therapy.

The first systemic approaches to preventing recurrence were hormonal. The general principle was removing estrogen before the menopause and replacing it afterwards. In effect, this was altering the hormonal milieu. The use of cytotoxic drugs came out of the success in treating leukemias and lymphomas in the 1960s, and followed on demonstrable success in inducing tumor regression using these agents in advanced breast cancer. With the identification of the estrogen and progesterone receptors in the 1970s, it became possible to stratify tumors into those likely to respond to hormone therapy and those unlikely to do so. As it happened, the preponderance of hormone-receptor-positive cancers were found in the postmenopausal population. Younger women were more likely to be hormone resistant, at least as measured by these tests. This lead to the generalization that chemotherapy is used most widely before the menopause, and hormonal manipulation is used after it.

More recently, the approach has been refined, and both hormonal and cytotoxic agents are used in both age groups, depending on individual prognostic information.

Hormonal manipulation

Beatson's landmark series of surgical castration in 1896 and, half a century later, the description of surgical adrenalectomy by Huggins and his colleagues were both empirical observations. Since then, a concentrated effort by endocrinologists and clinicians to understand and exploit these hormonal mechanisms has led to a dramatic fall in mortality from breast cancer over the last 15 years in both the UK and the USA.

Ovarian ablation. Interest in hormonal treatment has been reawakened. Two expected and one unexpected observation emerged from the overview of data up to 1985. The first was the expected predominance of chemotherapy benefit in premenopausal women with lesser benefit in the postmenopausal group, and the second was the mirror effect of tamoxifen, whose principal benefit comes after menopause. The surprise observation, however, was the meta-analysis of the mature data from a few relatively small trials of ovarian suppression (surgical castration or ovarian irradiation). The benefits of ovarian suppression were of the same order of magnitude as those achieved by cytotoxic chemotherapy.

These observations effectively established a research agenda for the next 15 years, which was driven by three fundamental questions.

- How does chemotherapy work in the adjuvant setting: by a direct cell-kill mechanism; by suppressing ovarian function; or in some other regulatory fashion?

- How should tissue predictive factors, such as estrogen and progesterone receptors, be used in addition to newer tests, such as *HER2-neu*?
- How can the use of two different therapies – hormones and cytotoxic agents – be optimized?

The original observation that ovarian suppression and chemotherapy each produced an improvement in disease-free survival in premenopausal women poses the question as to whether this effect was mediated indirectly by the same biochemical pathways. There are four sets of observations to support this hypothesis.

- It is recognized that cytotoxic chemotherapy will induce amenorrhea in a proportion of premenopausal women ranging from about 60% to nearly 100%, depending on age; the younger the woman, the greater the resistance to the castrating effect of cytotoxic drugs.
- The endocrinologic profile of a woman exposed to cytotoxic chemotherapy is similar to that of a castrated woman – in other words, estradiol levels fall and gonadotropin levels rise.
- There is now an extensive literature illustrating the fact that the induction of amenorrhea by adjuvant cytotoxic chemotherapy is in itself a prognostic factor. Those women who develop permanent amenorrhea fare better than those whose menstrual periods return during or after the completion of the course of treatment. This association is seen most clearly among women whose tumors express the estrogen/progesterone receptors.
- Data from clinical trials that have attempted a head-on comparison of endocrine therapy and chemotherapy suggest that ovarian suppression in ER+ve premenopausal women is equivalent to chemotherapy in terms of disease-free survival. The combination of a gonadotropin-releasing hormone (GnRH) analog plus tamoxifen is equivalent to chemotherapy plus tamoxifen if amenorrhea is achieved. Though the issues are complicated and doubtless uncertain, this raises the possibility that young women with ER+ve tumors who wish to remain fertile could be offered the choice of ovarian suppression including a GnRH agonist.

Tamoxifen has, for 20 years, been the benchmark antiestrogen; its therapeutic index and safety profile are truly remarkable. Treatment with this non-steroidal antiestrogen for between 2 and 5 years reduces the risk of death from breast cancer by 20–30% (Figure 6.1). It is believed to work by blocking the peripheral actions of estrogen (Figure 6.2). When estrogen binds to the surface estrogen receptors present in many tissues, a series of metabolic steps that stimulate proliferation are initiated at the nuclear level. Tamoxifen and other estrogen 'look-alike' compounds, such as raloxifene, bind to the same sites and block metabolic activity.

The improvement in mortality with tamoxifen persists for at least 10 years and occurs in women of all ages, although women aged over 50 years appear to derive the greatest benefit. The incidence of cancer in the opposite breast is also reduced by approximately 40% during tamoxifen treatment. In addition, serum levels of estrogen actually increase in response to tamoxifen in premenopausal women. Its mild estrogenic actions on tissues other than the breast, combined with different degrees of affinity between the drug and receptors in other tissues, explain the mixed agonist–antagonist response: thus, it may be associated with a reduced risk of coronary heart disease and osteoporosis, but also of occasional flares in advanced breast disease.

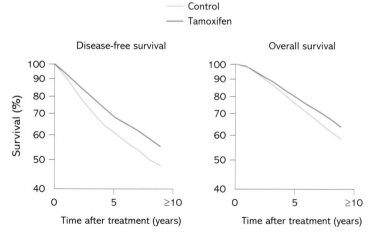

Figure 6.1 Treatment with tamoxifen, 20 mg/day, significantly improves disease-free and overall survival.

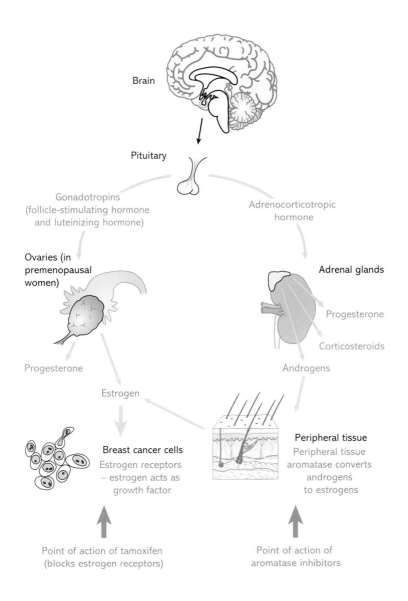

Figure 6.2 Tamoxifen and raloxifene act peripherally by binding to the surface estrogen receptors present in tissue, blocking estrogen itself from binding and initiating the series of steps leading to proliferation. In contrast, the aromatase inhibitors block production of estrogen.

The principal side effects are menopausal symptoms, such as hot flashes. There is, however, a small increase in the risk of endometrial cancer, which has been grossly overestimated in the media, and an increased risk of thromboembolic disorders. The increase in incidence does not exceed 1 case/1000 women treated with tamoxifen for 5 years, and the disease itself is almost always curable by hysterectomy. In general, the benefits of tamoxifen treatment outweigh the consequences of this small increase in risk.

The position of tamoxifen as the most important adjuvant therapy for early breast cancer is now clear.

- Tamoxifen has no role in the management of ER–ve cancers.
- Its benefit in premenopausal women is similar to that achieved in postmenopausal women.
- Its action is probably additive to that of chemotherapy.
- New evidence suggests that, if chemoendocrine therapy is used, tamoxifen should not be started until the chemotherapy has been completed.
- For every 1000 women treated with tamoxifen for 5 years, there would be 80 fewer breast cancer deaths set against one additional endometrial cancer death.

The hormone story is far from complete. It was observed that the small group of patients who were ER+ve/PR+ve and also positive for the growth factor receptor *HER2-neu* had an adverse response to tamoxifen. The research thus prompted suggests that there are in fact two estrogen-receptor actions, the familiar effect on the nucleus, in which the false transmitter blocks the downstream effects of estrogen, and a new point of action at the cell membrane. Here, tamoxifen acts like an estrogen and stimulates the overexpressed growth factor receptors to bypass the nucleus and promote cell proliferation. In animal studies, antibodies to the growth receptors (of which there are at least four) combined with tamoxifen provide dramatic, long reversals in tumor growth. This approach will appear in clinical trials within the next couple of years.

Aromatase inhibitors (AIs). 'Medical adrenalectomy' can be induced by the interruption of steroidogenesis at the level of the conversion of cholesterol to pregnenolone. It can achieve objective responses in metastatic breast cancer among women without ovarian function to a similar extent as a surgical adrenalectomy, and is thus more suitable for women who are a poor operative risk.

Recent developments in medical adrenalectomy have followed the discovery of AIs, which act by blocking aromatase, the enzyme that catalyzes the final and rate-limiting step in the synthesis of estrogens (Figure 6.2). Aromatase is expressed in non-ovarian tissues, such as muscle and fat, in both premenopausal and postmenopausal women. These non-ovarian tissues become the dominant sources of estrogen in postmenopausal women. Currently available AIs fall into two classes.

- The class I inhibitors bind aromatase irreversibly and have a steroidal structure (e.g. exemestane).
- The class II agents bind aromatase in a reversible manner and are nonsteroidal (e.g. anastrozole and letrozole).

Because of the specificity of its mode of action, this class of compound is remarkably non-toxic and therefore lends itself to the management of both early and advanced disease.

Both anastrozole and letrozole have been shown to be superior to megestrol acetate as second-line endocrine therapy after failure with tamoxifen. More importantly, however, both drugs have better efficacy and tolerability than tamoxifen as first-line therapy of locally advanced or metastatic disease in postmenopausal women with hormone-receptor-positive disease. However, the consequences for bone, heart and other organs of total estrogen withdrawal are likely to be greater than in the case of tamoxifen. In compensation, the risks of clotting and endometrial cancers are likely to be diminished. These agents are generally contraindicated in premenopausal women.

In early breast cancer, the third generation of oral AIs are ideal agents either to enhance the activity of tamoxifen or to replace it entirely in the adjuvant setting. A number of trials are exploring the role of both steroidal and non-steroidal agents used alone, sequentially or in combination with tamoxifen. These trials can be divided up into three groups:

- the comparison of an AI with tamoxifen as initial adjuvant therapy
- the switch to an AI after 2–3 years of tamoxifen compared with 5 years of tamoxifen
- the introduction of an AI after completing 5 years of tamoxifen compared with no further treatment.

ATAC (Arimidex, Tamoxifen Alone or in Combination) is the first trial to compare a new generation of AI with tamoxifen as initial treatment in postmenopausal women with early breast cancer. A unique feature of this trial was the inclusion of the combination arm, which evaluated the additive effects of the two drugs. In addition, the effects of both drugs on the endometrium, bone mineral density, bone markers and quality of life were assessed.

A total of 9366 postmenopausal patients with operable invasive breast cancer who had completed primary treatment were recruited into the trial, in 380 centers in 21 countries, between July 1996 and 2000. Patients were randomized to receive one of:

- tamoxifen, 20 mg, plus placebo
- anastrozole, 1 mg, plus placebo
- both active drugs.

At a relatively early stage, after about 4 years, anastrozole showed superior efficacy to tamoxifen, with a 17% relative risk reduction in disease-free survival in the intention-to-treat population, and a 19% improvement compared with the combination arm. The result was even better in women with hormone-sensitive (HR+ve) disease, in whom the relative risk reduction for anastrozole compared with tamoxifen was 27%. Surprisingly, the combination therapy group fared no better than the tamoxifen group and significantly worse than the anastrozole group; a possible explanation for this is that, in an estrogen-deprived environment, tamoxifen is 'seen' as an agonist, whereas in a normal estrogen-rich environment, tamoxifen can exert its classical antiestrogen effect. The combination arm was dropped and the trial continued with the two monotherapy arms. The results were updated at a median follow-up of over 5 years, when all but 8% of the patients had ceased therapy. These data were presented at the San Antonio Breast Cancer Symposium in December 2004. For the HR+ve group, anastrozole prevented one in four of the relapses seen in the tamoxifen-treated group, giving an absolute benefit of about 4% at 6 years of follow-up. Also for the first time, a significant reduction in distant recurrences was noted and a close to significant reduction in deaths from breast cancer.

Perhaps the most impressive result to date is the near-50% reduction in the incidence of contralateral invasive cancers with anastrozole compared with tamoxifen. Given that tamoxifen is associated with a 50% reduction in contralateral breast cancer over 5 years, if these trends persist, anastrozole has the potential to prevent (or delay) up to 75% of all cancers.

ATAC was powered to demonstrate 'equivalence' on the basis that anastrozole has a better tolerability profile than tamoxifen in patients with advanced disease. It could therefore be argued that, if this is the case in the adjuvant setting, anastrozole could become the treatment of choice. As it is, anastrozole already shows greater efficacy than tamoxifen after a relatively short follow-up period and, it could be argued, better tolerability; anastrozole is significantly less likely to contribute to hot flashes, vaginal discharge, vaginal bleeding, endometrial cancer, strokes and thromboembolic disease. Although endometrial cancer associated with exposure to tamoxifen is rare, fear of the disease means that most women with gynecological symptoms may be subjected to invasive investigations. Furthermore, at the update reported in December 2004, a fourfold reduction in hysterectomy rate was noted in the anastrozole group. Thus anastrozole, although more expensive in the short term, could in the long term save a great deal of unnecessary anxiety and healthcare costs. Formal health economic analyses have tended to support this assertion.

The disadvantages of anastrozole compared with tamoxifen are found in the contrast between women with chronic estrogen deprivation and women on a drug with weak agonist effect. Women receiving anastrozole are more likely to suffer from musculoskeletal problems, particularly a curious polyarthralgia, which seems to be a specific side effect of this class of compound. Its mechanism is obscure, but may be related to aromatase inhibition in the small muscles of the distal limbs. More serious, however, is the significant excess of fractures already observed in the anastrozole group; the problem appears to peak at about 3 years, but after 5 years the fracture rate seems to be the same as in the tamoxifen group. Whether this is a result of the protective effect of tamoxifen on bone compared with an untreated population, or whether it is due to estrogen deprivation because of aromatase inhibition, is speculative at this stage. Nevertheless, this side effect can be managed if anticipated. In women who are going to be treated with anastrozole, a bone density scan should be obtained at baseline and repeated at 12-monthly intervals. A variety of options can then be considered for women whose bone density starts to fall into the osteopenic range. For example, anastrozole could be withdrawn if the woman has been receiving treatment for more than about 3 years, or a bisphosphonate could be given, which might even reduce the risk of skeletal metastases as well as protecting the skeleton.

It is now the opinion of the ATAC trialists' group that anastrozole should replace tamoxifen as preferred therapy after primary surgery for postmenopausal women with HR+ve disease, a view shared by the authors of this book (one of whom [MB] was involved in the trial) and endorsed by the new American Society of Clinical Oncology (ASCO) guidelines published in January 2005 in the *Journal of Clinical Oncology*. The guidelines recommend that optimal adjuvant therapy should now include use of an AI to reduce risk of tumor recurrence.

Trials comparing tamoxifen for 5 years with 2–3 years of tamoxifen followed by a switch to an AI. So far three trials of a very similar design have reported on this policy, one using exemestane (the BIG IES trial) and two using anastrozole, a small Italian trial and a large combined Austrian and German trial (ITA and ABCSG/ARNO).

In the BIG IES study, treatment with tamoxifen for 5 years was compared with tamoxifen for 2–3 years followed by exemestane to achieve a total of 5 years of adjuvant hormonal treatment. This multinational trial involving 4742 patients demonstrated a 32% reduction in recurrence risk corresponding to an absolute benefit of 4.7% in disease-free survival. Predictably, the short median follow-up of 30.6 months did not enable a survival difference or an increased incidence of long-term adverse effects, such as bone fracture, to be shown.

The ITA trial was of similar design, although using anastrozole as the AI, and it demonstrated similar results. The ABCSG/ARNO trial, also using anastrozole, was presented for the first time in December 2004. Patients in the study group were switched from tamoxifen to the AI at two years. The striking finding here was a near-40% reduction in both event-free survival and distant recurrence. Interestingly, there was little difference in gynecological problems between the two arms, probably because all the patients had already been exposed to 2 years of tamoxifen, during which time most of these symptoms arise.

National Cancer Institute of Canada Clinical Trials Group Intergroup trial MA17. In this trial, women who were alive and symptom-free after taking tamoxifen for 5 years were randomized to receive placebo or letrozole for a further 5 years. The trial was aborted (prematurely, some think) because of a significant improvement in disease-free survival in the letrozole group. These results generated much excitement, being the first to suggest that the natural history of breast cancer can be favorably perturbed beyond 5 years of tamoxifen. In addition, an update of this study presented to ASCO in May 2004 reported that for the node-positive group a significant improvement in overall survival had emerged.

Selection of the best option. A choice of adjuvant endocrine therapy is now available for postmenopausal patients with hormone-sensitive disease. If tamoxifen is specifically contraindicated, for example because of a previous history of thromboembolic disease, an AI should be considered. However, the new data from ATAC may persuade many oncologists that it is now appropriate to start with the AI in the first place.

With regard to switching from tamoxifen to an AI after 2–3 years of tamoxifen, the results of three trials reported late in 2004 all suggest that this might be a wise choice. The same might also be said for starting an AI after completing 5 years of tamoxifen therapy. While the experts will continue to debate the most appropriate scheduling of tamoxifen and an AI for some time to come, there seems little doubt that the drug that has served us so well for 20 years may soon be past its 'sell-by date'. However, for the premenopausal woman, and in the developing world, where cost issues make any aspect of cancer care a problem, tamoxifen still has a long life ahead.

Chemotherapy

Adjuvant chemotherapy as a strategy is more than 30 years old. The original premises were extrapolations of experience in advanced disease and began with the assumption that, if cytotoxic drugs were effective when the tumor volume was large, an even better result might be obtained when the volume was microscopic. This is somewhat countered by an important corollary to the log-cell-kill hypothesis that underlies modern cytotoxic chemotherapy. This states that for every doubling of dose, another log-kill of target cells takes place. The corollary is that it is impossible to kill the last cell!

From the outset the challenge has been to determine who to treat and for how long, and the timing with respect to other treatments. This was made more difficult because, by definition, there was nothing to see or visibly follow. The only evidence came from clinical trials and population-based studies; those who were treated had fewer recurrences and, as a group, lived longer.

The public perception that chemotherapy is very toxic is a result of early experience with these drugs. Nowadays, side effects are sufficiently manageable that almost all adjuvant chemotherapy is provided on an outpatient basis, and many patients are able to achieve substantial activity levels during the weeks and months of treatment.

Timing. The assumption has always been that chemotherapy should be initiated as close to the time of surgery as possible. The neoadjuvant concept advances this to encompass the operative period.

Drugs. The drugs used will depend on the prognosis, the patient's comorbidities and lifestyle, and the experience of the treating specialist. A combination of several different types of drug is usually given (Table 6.1), which has the benefit of providing different points of metabolic attack, while minimizing toxicities.

TABLE 6.1

Common adjuvant chemotherapy regimens

Regimen	Agents	Number of cycles	Cycle length (days)	Treatment duration (months)
CMF*	Cyclophosphamide[§] Methotrexate Fluorouracil	6	28	6
CEF[†]	Cyclophosphamide[§] Epirubicin Fluorouracil	6	28	6
AC[†]	Doxorubicin Cyclophosphamide[¶]	4	21	3
FAC[†]	Fluorouracil Doxorubicin Cyclophosphamide[¶]	6	21	4–6 (how quickly treatment can be administered depends on ability to tolerate side effects)
FEC[†]	Fluorouracil Epirubicin Cyclophosphamide[¶]	6	21	4–6 (how quickly treatment can be administered depends on ability to tolerate side effects)
AC+T[‡]	Doxorubicin Cyclophosphamide[¶] Followed by paclitaxel alone	4 4	21	6
AC+T + recom-binant G-CSF[‡]	Doxorubicin Cyclophosphamide[¶] Followed by paclitaxel alone	4 4	14 (dose dense)	5
TAC[‡]	Docetaxel Adriamycin Cyclophosphamide[¶]	6	21	4–6 (how quickly treatment can be administered depends on ability to tolerate side effects)

*This regimen has been in use the longest and has become the baseline standard.
[†]These regimens include an anthracycline and are considered more intensive.
[‡]These regimens include a taxane, which increases toxicity; they are considered the most aggressive regimens.
[§]Cyclophosphamide administered as a tablet.
[¶]Cyclophosphamide administered into a vein.
G-CSF, granulocyte colony-stimulating factor.

Cyclophosphamide is an alkylating agent related to nitrogen mustard, but less toxic and far easier to handle. It has been a mainstay of adjuvant therapy for breast cancer from the outset. Its side effects include nausea and vomiting, bone-marrow suppression, hair loss when given in large doses, and sterile hemorrhagic cystitis if high levels of urinary output are not maintained. Myelodysplastic syndromes, including acute leukemias, are seen very occasionally.

Methotrexate and 5-fluorouracil are antimetabolites, also of long standing. Their side effects are subtler and more varied, and include diarrhea, rashes, watery eyes and, in high doses, bone-marrow suppression.

Anthracyclines, including adriamycin, epirubicin and mitoxantrone, are powerful DNA intercalators employed in mid-range and aggressive regimens. As single agents, they are the most effective drugs in advanced breast cancer. They were not used until the efficacy of the adjuvant strategy with alkylating drugs was established, because of concerns about their greater propensity to bone-marrow suppression, rare myelodysplastic syndromes and leukemias, total alopecia, and nausea and vomiting. The anthracyclines also carry a distinct risk of cardiotoxicity; pathologically, a progressive random degradation of myocardial cells is observed, leading to pump failure. The long-term consequences for the heart are unknown, but the prevailing view is that, in patients without pre-existing myocardial compromise, these drugs offer benefit considerably in excess of the toxic risk.

Taxanes, including paclitaxel and docetaxel, are spindle inhibitors. Their major side effects are peripheral neuropathies and acute reactions. The taxanes seem to be effective in advanced disease, even in tumors resistant to anthracyclines. They are just emerging from the clinical trials setting towards becoming an 'established' adjuvant therapy.

Monoclonal antibodies are the newest class of drug, and trastuzumab is the first 'proof of concept' drug. Trastuzumab attaches to *HER2-neu*, which is one of several epidermal growth factor receptors in a family of transmembrane proteins involved in the regulation of cell proliferation. It is often overexpressed in breast cancers so, by blocking the receptor, trastuzumab inhibits proliferation. As a single agent, it has a modest effect with a response rate of about

20% in advanced disease, but it seems to act synergistically when combined with other agents. However, trastuzumab has significant cardiac toxicity and, at present, its role in adjuvant treatment should be restricted to clinical trials.

In advanced disease, trastuzumab, especially when combined with other effective agents such as the anthracyclines or taxanes, can provide good and occasionally sustained responses. An emerging strategy is to induce a maximal response with combination treatment, and maintain it with the antibody.

Small molecules. Our advancing molecular regulatory understanding of breast cancer has stimulated a broad attack on defective pathways. One example, a tyrosine kinase inhibitor called gefitinib (Iressa), has come to market for lung cancer and shows some promise in animal models of breast cancer.

Dose and duration. The dose and duration of treatment has been the subject of a long-simmering debate. The original adjuvant treatments, with the notable exception of the perioperative use of cyclophosphamide as a single agent, were used for up to 2 years. Subsequently, the trend has been to shorten the duration of treatment to 6 months, based on data from clinical trials. This trend led to the concept of dose intensity and the suggestion that total dose was not as important as the dose per treatment. An increasingly controversial series of studies of ever-higher doses followed, leading ultimately to trials of such intensity that rescue strategies for bone-marrow transplant were required as part of the treatment. When objective data (all negative) were finally obtained from clinical trials, the strategy was abandoned.

The concept of dose density (total dose in a defined time), as distinct from dose intensity, is attracting some attention. The premise is that supportive therapies such as erythropoietin and granulocyte colony-stimulating factor enable shorter intervals between doses and may thus improve efficacy. One trial result from the US Cancer and Leukemia Group B, of about 3.5 years follow-up, offers some provocative evidence. Patients tolerate the treatment well, but it is very expensive. Ongoing trials bear watching.

Thus, the questions of dose, intensity and duration are still not resolved. The uncertain mechanism of action gives grounds for debate. If cell kill is what makes the difference, then intensity and exposure to multiple agents will be important. If, on the other hand, alterations in the tumor–host milieu or regulatory mechanisms are at the heart of the matter, it is likely that longer-lasting, less intense strategies will come to predominate. Small molecules, such as highly targeted proteins, and antiangiogenesis factors (including cyclo-oxygenase [COX]-2 inhibitors) seem to cure mice; the question now is whether they cure people. There is enough clinical evidence, albeit anecdotal, to make this an area of intense exploration. We are coming to understand that a late-stage tumor is not simply an older and bigger early-stage cancer, so a drug development strategy which requires efficacy in the advanced setting before adjuvant studies can be considered is not appropriate for this class of agent, unlike the classic cytotoxic drugs.

Sequencing. Surgery, hormonal treatment and chemotherapy interact. The sequence to date has been driven by practice and convention as much as by science. Surgery has come first. More recently, neoadjuvant approaches have been tried. Four observations underlie modern, scientifically disciplined approaches to combining surgery, radiation and systemic treatments in early-stage breast cancer.

- Breast cancer is a systemic disease from the outset. Therefore, local control is likely to have only a small effect on overall outcome. A recent meta-analysis largely confirms this, with the important caveats that radiation is required for those opting for lumpectomy, and that failure to achieve local control adds about 4% to mortality at 15–20 years (see page 77).
- Removal of the primary tumor in animal models leads to a transient burst of proliferation in metastases, especially small occult ones. The 40–60% reduction in recurrence rates with adjuvant systemic therapies as currently given is partial confirmation. The fact that neoadjuvant treatments do not improve overall or disease-free survival despite pathological complete remission at the primary site in as much as 26% of the study populations may be equally important supportive evidence.

- Cytotoxic drugs kill proliferating cells more effectively than they kill resting cells. The actions of hormones and their antagonists, receptor-targeted antibodies and regulatory pathway drugs depend less on the cell cycle.
- The current practice of withholding hormones (which inhibit proliferation) until chemotherapy is complete will have to be closely watched. It seems a trifle counterintuitive to hold back the more effective treatment for HR+ve patients until the less effective one has been given.

  Three nested questions will have to be tested clinically.
- As the range of regulatory drugs and their requisite markers expand, the role of cytotoxics will have to be retested.
- The value of targeting the postlumpectomy proliferative burst will have to be reconsidered.
- We need to know how important tumor heterogeneity is, and how it comes about: spontaneously or driven by treatment?

Putting it all together for patients

The decision to offer adjuvant therapy is complex along three axes:

- the best treatment in the abstract
- treatment interactions with comorbidities in a particular patient
- the patient's preference.

There are some very general rules of thumb as starting points.

- Hormone therapy reduces the proportionate risk of recurrence by about 40% in ER+ve/PR+ve patients.
- Chemotherapy reduces the proportionate risk by about 33%, with CMF being the baseline standard. Anthracyclines add a further 5–10%, and, if early data are reliable, the taxanes perhaps another 5–10%.
- Chemotherapy works best for HR–ve patients.
- Combining chemotherapy and hormones has an approximately 15% added proportionate benefit.
- The issue for an individual patient is absolute risk, not relative risk, as outlined in Chapter 2, so population estimates of proportionate benefit must be converted to estimates of absolute benefit for the individual, which can then be set against treatment risk.

Key points – adjuvant therapy

- Both hormonal and chemotherapeutic adjuvant treatment decrease the risk of recurrence by about 33%. The field is changing, and combined approaches are increasingly common.
- The efficacy of very-high-dose chemotherapy, including bone-marrow transplantation, remains unproven.
- Aromatase inhibitors show great promise in clinical trials, and may come to replace antiestrogens, such as tamoxifen.
- Well-designed and managed clinical trials remain the preferred context for treatment.

In order to help with individual decision making, Peter Ravdin, at the University of Texas San Antonio, has devised a program (available free at www.adjuvantonline.com) that uses algorithms derived from clinical trials data to calculate the proportionate and, more importantly, absolute benefit of a range of adjuvant interventions in individual cases (Figure 6.3). It is intended for healthcare professionals, but the output includes a graphic for the patient.

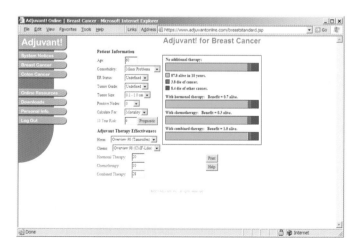

Figure 6.3 The 'Adjuvant!' online program calculates the risks and benefits of interventions (www.adjuvantonline.com). Reproduced with permission.

Side effects. Chemotherapy is associated with a number of side effects (Table 6.2). Although hair loss is the most common concern of patients, complete alopecia is rare except with doxorubicin. Wigs can be supplied if the loss is very noticeable, and the hair regrows at the end of treatment. In practice, fatigue and lethargy are the most troublesome side effects in 80% of patients. Nausea and vomiting can be controlled in most patients by antiemetic agents. Infertility occurs in up to 40% of patients, and this possibility should be discussed before treatment begins if the woman wishes to have children in the future. It is important to balance these side effects against the overall benefit to the patient, taking into account the risk of recurrence (or likelihood of response in advanced disease), comorbidities and the individual's particular concerns about the consequences of these side effects.

TABLE 6.2

Side effects of adjuvant chemotherapy for breast cancer

- Fatigue and lethargy
- Alopecia (temporary)
- Nausea and vomiting
- Risk of infection
- Oral mucositis
- Diarrhea
- Infertility
- Weight gain
- Consequences of premature menopause
- Leukemia and myelodysplastic disorders
- Peripheral neuropathy
- Allergic and vascular reactions with taxanes

Key references

American College of Obstetricians and Gynecologists. Tamoxifen and endometrial cancer. *Obstet Gynecol* 2000;95:1C–3C.

ATAC Trials group. Anastrozole alone or in combination with tamoxifen versus tamoxifen alone for adjuvant treatment of post menopausal women with early-stage breast cancer. Results of the ATAC (Arimidex, Tamoxifen Alone or in Combination) trial efficacy and safety update analyses. *Cancer* 2003;98:1802–10.

Baum M, Buzdar AU, Cuzick J et al. Anastrozole alone or in combination with tamoxifen versus tamoxifen alone for adjuvant treatment of postmenopausal women with early breast cancer: first results of the ATAC randomised trial. *Lancet* 2002;360:2131–9.

Coombes RC, Hall E, Gibson LJ et al. A randomized trial of exemestane after two or three years of tamoxifen therapy in postmenopausal women with primary breast cancer. *N Engl J Med* 2004;350:1081–92.

Early Breast Cancer Trialists' Collaborative Group. *A Systematic Over-view of All Available Randomized Trials of Adjuvant Endocrine and Cytotoxic Therapy*. Oxford: Oxford University Press, 1990.

Early Breast Cancer Trialists' Collaborative Group. Systemic treatment of early breast cancer by hormonal, cytotoxic, or immune therapy; 133 randomised trials involving 31 000 recurrences and 24 000 deaths among 75 000 women. *Lancet* 1992;339:1–5.

Early Breast Cancer Trialists' Collaborative Group. Ovarian ablation in early breast cancer: overview of randomised trials. *Lancet* 1996;348:1189–96.

Early Breast Cancer Trialists' Collaborative Group. Tamoxifen for early breast cancer: an overview of the randomised trials. *Lancet* 1998; 351:1451–67.

Fisher B, Dignam J, Bryant J et al. Five versus more than five years of tamoxifen therapy for breast cancer patients with negative lymph nodes and estrogen receptor-positive tumors. *J Natl Cancer Inst* 1996;88:1529–42.

Goss PE, Ingle JN, Martino S et al. A randomized trial of letrozole in postmenopausal women after five years of tamoxifen therapy for early stage breast cancer. *N Engl J Med* 2003;349:1793–802.

Howell A, Cuzick J, Baum M et al. Results of the ATAC (Arimidex, Tamoxifen, Alone or in Combination) trial after completion of 5 years' adjuvant treatment for breast cancer. *Lancet* 2005;365:60–2.

Huggins C, Bergenstal DM. Inhibition of human mammary and prostatic cancer by adrenalectomy. *Cancer Res* 1952;12:134–41.

Meier CR. Tamoxifen and risk of idiopathic venous thromboembolism. *Br J Clin Pharmacol* 1998;45:608–12.

McDonald CC, Alexander FE, Whyte BW et al. Cardiac and vascular morbidity in women receiving adjuvant tamoxifen in a randomized trial. *BMJ* 1995;311:977–80.

Nabholtz JM, Buzdar A, Pollak M et al. Anastrozole is superior to tamoxifen as first-line therapy for advanced breast cancer in postmenopausal women – results of a North American multicenter randomized trial. *J Clin Oncol* 2000;18:3758–67.

Winer EP, Hudis C, Burstein HJ et al. American Society of Clinical Oncology technology assessment on the use of aromatase inhibitors as adjuvant therapy for postmenopausal women with hormone receptor-positive breast cancer: status report 2004. *J Clin Oncol* 2005;23:619–29.

This extremely complex issue can be very confusing, given the claims and counterclaims in newspapers and scientific journals. Every time a study is reported in the press, women are made anxious; of those, some may abandon their hormone replacement therapy (HRT) without consultation, while others will consult their physician in the hope of receiving a simple answer.

At issue is whether the estrogen in HRT can initiate or accelerate the development of breast cancer. Estrogen is a steroid hormone produced principally in the ovaries of premenopausal women, but still present, at lower levels, in postmenopausal women. It is prescribed, sometimes in conjunction with progesterone, to alleviate menopausal symptoms and maintain bone density.

The first piece of evidence implicating estrogens in the development of breast cancer is that the disease is very uncommon in men; it does occur, but more than 100 times less frequently than in women. More direct evidence comes from the fact that a very early menopause or surgical castration for ovarian disease is protective for breast cancer, whereas a late menopause (i.e. a prolonged natural exposure to estrogen) is associated with an increased risk. After the menopause, estrogens are produced in the fatty tissues of the body by the enzyme aromatase. Postmenopausal women with a lot of body fat have higher levels of estrogen than those with little body fat, and are at greater risk of breast cancer. Furthermore, both the antiestrogen tamoxifen and the drug anastrozole, which switches off the production of estrogen in postmenopausal women, reduce the risk of breast cancer and are being investigated in trials for the prevention of the disease.

Of less importance, in the authors' opinion, is the extensive literature on animal experiments that support this thesis. It should, however, be noted that, certainly in humans, the culprit could equally well be progesterone as estrogen; this will be considered later.

There are two scenarios that must be kept separate when considering HRT and breast cancer:

- the risk of developing breast cancer after long-term exposure to HRT in women who have not had the disease
- the risk of recurrence in women taking HRT who have previously been treated for breast cancer.

It is also essential to make a distinction between combined HRT, which includes progesterone as well as estrogen, and estrogen replacement therapy alone. The former is prescribed when a woman still has her uterus, because unopposed estrogen is associated with an increased incidence of endometrial cancer. Women who have had a hysterectomy are usually prescribed estrogen replacement therapy alone.

Quality of evidence

It is important to consider the quality of the evidence linking HRT with breast cancer risk. There are broadly two types of research design.

- In a randomized controlled trial, women are allocated completely at random to receive either an active compound or a placebo. Trials of this type are more able to detect a true effect.
- In an observational study, women are given HRT and monitored long term, and the incidence of harmful and beneficial effects are then compared with a matched population. This type of study is open to considerable bias.

Sadly, no initial randomized controlled trials to establish safety and efficacy were performed before the widespread adoption of HRT about 30 years ago. This would be unthinkable today, but as a result of what might be considered a natural experiment, thousands of women were followed up. The data obtained were, however, often misleading. For example, for a long time, it was thought that the use of HRT would protect against heart attacks and Alzheimer's disease; this is no longer thought to be the case. At the same time, there is unequivocal evidence that HRT improves quality of life, reduces the incidence of hot flashes and night sweats, and protects the skeleton from osteoporosis. The suggestion that long-term exposure to HRT is linked to an increased risk of breast cancer is not new, but the estimates of this risk have always been unreliable.

Recent studies

The HRT debate has moved rapidly within the last 12 months or so, following the publication of three landmark papers.

The Heart and Estrogen/progestin Replacement Study (HERS) involved nearly 1300 women who had already experienced a heart attack. Combined continuous HRT was found *not* to prevent additional heart attacks, as was originally thought from observational studies. HRT was also associated with more cases of venous thromboembolic disease. However, the mortality from all causes was the same in both groups. The women taking HRT had fewer hot flashes, less vaginal dryness and fewer episodes of depression (the so-called climacteric syndrome).

The Women's Health Initiative (WHI) study was of a similar design to HERS, but involved women who had no history of heart problems. The women were randomized to receive either combined continuous HRT (estrogen and progesterone) or estrogen therapy alone. The first component of the study involving 8500 women receiving combined continuous HRT was stopped, and the results were published, when the independent data monitoring committee considered it unethical to continue. The average age of the women in this study was 63 years and follow-up was about 5 years. In addition to establishing the relative risk, absolute numbers of important medical events were described, which can be helpful to women trying to decide whether or not to take HRT. If 10 000 women took combination HRT, for each year there would be:

- 7 additional cases of heart attack
- 8 additional cases of stroke
- 8 additional cases of pulmonary embolism
- 8 additional cases of invasive breast cancer
- 6 fewer cases of hip fracture.

Curiously, a reduction in the risk of colon cancer that almost counterbalanced the additional risk of breast cancer was also noted.

The Million Women study, unlike HERS and the WHI study, was observational rather than randomized. The study involved 1 million women who accepted an invitation for mammographic screening. The women were questioned about their use of HRT, and this was then related to the subsequent development of breast cancer. The headline result was that the women who had taken combined HRT had a relative risk of breast cancer of 2.0 after an average follow-up period of about 2.5 years. For those on estrogen replacement alone, the relative risk was about 1.5. Translated into absolute numbers, combined HRT would contribute an extra 20 cases/10 000 women/year and estrogen replacement therapy alone an extra 10 cases/10 000 women/year.

This study has been subjected to a lot of criticism as it only involved women who accepted an invitation for screening. These women may not have been representative of the total population and may have included more women with a family history of breast cancer than an unselected group. Furthermore, HRT makes mammograms extremely difficult to interpret, and it is possible that these cancers were present at the time of initial screening, but overlooked, and then ultimately diagnosed 1–2 years later.

Harm–benefit analysis. Bearing in mind that most women take HRT to improve their quality of life by preventing hot flashes and night sweats, the harm–benefit analysis can be judged a close call.

It should be noted that, although the WHI study revealed eight additional breast cancers/10 000 women/year, the cancers tended to be of a more favorable, less aggressive type, and an excess of deaths from breast cancer has not yet been seen. It must be emphasized that an increased incidence of disease does not automatically translate into an increase in deaths from the disease.

Another factor that must be considered is that both HERS and the WHI study used combination therapy, and it remains just as likely that the culprit is the progesterone component as the estrogen component. This suggestion has now been supported by the results from the estrogen-only arm of the WHI study, which was recently closed because of a slight increase in the incidence of stroke. Notably, *no* adverse effects in terms of either heart disease or breast cancer were seen. Bearing in mind that estrogens protect against osteoporosis, many would argue that the as yet unpublished data on the 'slight increased risk of stroke' would be more than compensated for by reduction in fracture rate and enhanced quality of life.

For women with intolerable acute menopausal symptoms, established osteoporosis or a family history of osteoporosis, HRT must still be considered an option under the guidance of a gynecologist. It is also worth considering whether combined therapy should be abandoned even for women with an intact uterus, as the risk of unopposed estrogen inducing endometrial cancer is less than the risk of inducing breast cancer with the combined preparation.

High-risk families

The decision about HRT is much more difficult for those women with a poor family history of breast cancer. A genetic predisposition can be suspected when the pedigree demonstrates that every other female member has developed breast cancer or ovarian cancer. The suspicion is increased if the individual's age at onset of the cancer is under 40 years or if a relative had cancer affecting both breasts. Occasionally, these families also include a male relative with breast cancer. For such women, the risk of developing breast cancer might be ten times that of the normal population and, if they are tested and found to carry the mutated gene, the risk of developing breast cancer in the future is 60–70%. Furthermore, the breast cancers that develop in such families tend to be more aggressive and insensitive to hormones.

The issue for women with a suspected genetic predisposition to breast cancer is not about HRT, but whether or not they should consider preventative mastectomy or even preventative oophorectomy (castration). Such women should be referred to specialist clinics with onward referral to a clinical geneticist if indicated. It must, however, be emphasized that such families are very rare and account for less than 5% of all breast cancers.

The woman with one first-degree relative with breast cancer (e.g. mother or sister) is much more commonly encountered. Indeed, the impact on a woman's risk of developing breast cancer based on a family history is a common reason for referral to breast-care clinics. In order to demonstrate how the risk is calculated, the simplest example will be used in which a woman is worried because her mother has just been diagnosed with breast cancer at the age of 50. In addition, the woman has just turned 30 years of age and has not yet had any children. Taking these two risk factors together gives a relative risk of 2, that is, twice the normal risk of developing breast cancer. Bearing in mind that this woman is 30 and that the normal risk is 1 cancer/1000 women/year, then twice that risk is 2 cancers/1000 women/year, which on aggregate is less than 5% until she reaches the menopause (2 cancers/ 1000 women/year for 20 years is 40 cancers/1000 women, or 4%). After the woman reaches 50 years of age, her background risk grows to twice this over the next decade and, in the worst-case scenario, the addition of combined HRT again doubles the risk. The risk now reaches 8% on aggregate over the decade (4 cancers/1000 women/year, doubled by HRT, over 10 years), which might be considered unacceptable in spite of all the assumptions and uncertainties. At this point, alternatives to HRT have to be considered (see page 108).

HRT during or after treatment for breast cancer

The conventional wisdom is that estrogens are contraindicated in women affected by breast cancer. As a consequence, many women suffering from acute menopausal symptoms, which are sometimes provoked by the breast cancer treatment itself, are denied access to an effective source of relief.

There are, however, two paradoxes that must be considered. First, in the days before the 'antiestrogen' tamoxifen, high doses of estrogen were often prescribed for advanced breast cancer with remarkable results. Secondly, tamoxifen is a very effective drug in premenopausal women with early breast cancer, leading to the same prolongation of life and cure rates as among postmenopausal women. In younger women, however, tamoxifen actually induces extremely high levels of estrogen by blocking the feedback mechanism in the hypothalamus and pituitary. Despite this, the results with tamoxifen are unimpaired, so it would appear that high levels of estrogens in the circulation do not necessarily inhibit the benefits of antiestrogens.

There is a need for randomized controlled trials to compare HRT with placebo in women affected by breast cancer. Three clinical trials are now under way: one in the UK, and two in Sweden. Only the results of the Swedish HABITS (hormonal replacement therapy after breast cancer – is it safe?) trial have been published to date.

HABITS trial. This trial has provided the first good-quality evidence that HRT in the early years after breast cancer treatment can indeed hasten the appearance of breast cancer recurrences. The study involved 434 women suffering from climacteric symptoms, half of whom received HRT, while the other half acted as controls. On average, most women entered the study 2.5 years after treatment for their disease. About half of all the women had been on HRT before diagnosis. The study was interrupted 5 years after it started as it became clear that the women in the HRT group had a significant increase in the risk of recurrence.

At the time of analysis, 26 women in the HRT group had developed a new breast cancer event compared with 7 in the control group. The bulk of the difference was in the patients with hormone-receptor-positive tumors, but it seemed to make little difference whether or not they were taking tamoxifen. Because of the relative immaturity of these data, it is not yet clear whether the risk applies equally to the combined HRT and the estrogen-alone treatments.

It is likely that when the information from the other two studies (which will probably be aborted as a result of HABITS) is added to the data already available, the estimate of risk will be refined, but it still leaves tough choices for women with hormone-receptor-positive tumors suffering from hot flashes, night sweats and depression.

Alternatives to HRT

Natural products and alternative medicine. A large number of natural products and alternative interventions must be considered 'unproven'. Most of the products on the market are, however, believed to be safe, even though their efficacy is based on anecdote alone. Among the most popular of these alternatives are extract of red clover and vegetables rich in phytoestrogens.

Raloxifene, a selective estrogen-receptor modulator (SERM), is a compound similar to tamoxifen. It is an important drug in the management of osteoporosis and also appears to have a protective effect against the development of breast cancer. However, it has no beneficial effect on climacteric symptoms.

Tibolone is a steroid molecule that, in theory, matches the ideal product profile for the treatment of climacteric complaints and the prevention of bone loss in postmenopausal women. It undoubtedly has favorable effects on bone, vaginal dryness, hot flashes, night sweats, mood and sexual wellbeing, without stimulating the endometrium or the breast. It is currently widely used, particularly for women with a poor family history of breast cancer.

A recent survey of all the available literature shows no indication of an increased risk of breast cancer with tibolone, except for the Million Women study. In that study, a small increased relative risk was seen in women who had previously used tibolone. However, as this drug is favored by women who already have an increased risk of breast cancer because of a family history, this finding, in the authors' opinion, can be discounted.

Three large-scale, randomized trials are currently comparing tibolone with placebo with respect to effects on heart, bone and risk of breast cancer. In particular, the LIBERATE study aims to look at over 2000 women who have previously been treated for breast cancer to determine whether tibolone is associated with an increased risk of recurrence of breast cancer. However, in the face of uncertainty, tibolone, 2.5 mg daily, appears a reasonable option, at least in the short term, pending the publication of the results of the LIBERATE study.

Antidepressants. There are anecdotal reports that selective serotonin-reuptake inhibitors (SSRIs) relieve hot flashes. Two of these agents, venlafaxine and paroxetine hydrochloride, have recently been evaluated in properly designed randomized controlled trials, and the early results look encouraging.

Key points – hormone replacement therapy and breast cancer

- The climacteric syndrome impairs the quality of life for women with or without breast cancer.
- Estrogen replacement therapy (ERT) is the most effective of several options for dealing with this problem.
- Though the role of hormone therapy is under intense scrutiny, it is clear that the risk–benefit ratio is less favorable than earlier thought.
- Hormone replacement therapy (HRT) is linked to an increased incidence of breast cancer, raising breast cancer risk proportionate to an individual's pre-existing risk.
- The roles of estrogen and progesterone are not clear, but it seems likely that progesterone rather than estrogen is the culprit.
- The published trials used larger doses than currently advocated.
- Such data as exist suggest that HRT less than 3 years after breast cancer raises the recurrence risk.
- Doctors and patients together should weigh up the undoubted benefits of ERT against the theoretical hazards of HRT rather than prohibiting a life-enhancing intervention.

Key references

Barlow DH, Wren BG. *Fast Facts – Menopause*, 2nd edn. Oxford: Health Press, 2005.

Grady D, Herrington D, Bittner V et al. Cardiovascular disease outcomes during 6.8 years of hormone therapy: Heart and Estrogen/progestin Replacement Study follow-up (HERS II). *JAMA* 2002;288:49–57.

Holmberg L, Anderson H. HABITS (hormonal replacement therapy after breast cancer – is it safe?), a randomised comparison: trial stopped. *Lancet* 2004;363:453–5.

Loprinzi CL, Kugler JW, Sloan JA. Venlafaxine in management of hot flashes in survivors of breast cancer: a randomised controlled trial. *Lancet* 2000;356:2059–63.

Million Women Study Collaborators. Breast cancer and hormone-replacement therapy: the Million Women Study. *Lancet* 2003; 362:419–27.

Minelli C, Abrams KR, Sutton AJ et al. Benefits and harms associated with hormone replacement therapy: clinical decision analysis. *BMJ* 2004;328:371–5.

Powledge TM. NIH terminates WHI oestrogen-only study. *Lancet* 2004; 363:870.

Rossouw JE, Anderson GL, Prentice RL et al. Risks and benefits of estrogen plus progestin in healthy postmenopausal women: principal results from the Women's Health Initiative randomized controlled trial. *JAMA* 2002;288:321–33.

Stearns V, Isaacs C, Rowland J et al. A pilot trial assessing the efficacy of paroxetine hydrochloride (Paxil) in controlling hot flashes in breast cancer survivors. *Ann Oncol* 2000; 11:17–22.

Follow-up

The conventional teaching is that patients who have completed primary and systemic therapy for breast cancer should be followed up until relapse or death from the disease or intercurrent illness. In addition to clinical examination to detect local regional recurrence or contralateral disease, these patients often undergo regular radiological and serological examinations to search for occult metastases. These examinations may include a chest radiograph, an ultrasound scan of the liver, skeletal scintigraphy and measurement of tumor markers, such as carbohydrate antigen 15-3 (CA 15-3) or carcinoembryonic antigen (CEA).

This convention has, however, been challenged in recent years. On the basis of several carefully controlled studies in Europe and North America, it is now appreciated that most local or distant metastases present themselves between the routine follow-up intervals and that the 'lead time' achieved by a search for asymptomatic distant disease is of little value, as it contributes nothing to the survival or quality of life of the patient. A less interventional approach involves clinical follow-up with history and examinations every 3 months for about 2 years, subsequently extending the interval between visits. An annual chest radiograph, complete blood count, measurement of serum calcium levels and liver function tests provide a prudent middle ground. For this approach to work, however, it is vital that the patient should be well informed and present promptly should symptoms develop. A number of randomized controlled trials have been proposed, or are in progress, to compare intensive and minimal follow-up. Outcome measures include patient satisfaction, quality of life and, in particular, the presence or absence of uncontrolled local recurrence in the conserved breast.

Mammography. The role of mammography in follow-up is somewhat controversial. Following breast conservation surgery, many surgeons seem to lack the courage of their convictions, and obsessively check and recheck the preserved breast clinically and radiologically. Not surprisingly, this leads to a state of chronic anxiety for the patient. Furthermore, mammography is not a valuable imaging technique after breast conservation surgery because the scarring that may persist for 1–2 years cannot be distinguished from the stellate appearance of a carcinoma.

Clinicians and patients alike have to be reassured that the risk of local relapse within the retained breast is similar to the risk of a contralateral breast cancer, which is about 7% over 10 years. Furthermore, there is no evidence that local recurrence in the ipsilateral breast is directly associated with excess mortality. The relative risk of dying of a contralateral breast cancer depends on the recurrence risk associated with the original tumor. It may be extremely small when compared with the risk of death from the original disease. For this reason a policy of biennial mammography, for example, might be a reasonable compromise, but the routine use of tumor markers or imaging tests in the search for distant metastases cannot be endorsed. None of these tests has a high specificity, and the patient can therefore often suffer false alarms. Moreover, even if the results are truly positive for asymptomatic metastases, this merely provides the patient with 6 months' notice of impending death, during which time the reintroduction of systemic therapy is of unproven value.

Rehabilitation

Patients undergoing surgery for primary breast cancer require rehabilitation to address the physical and psychological consequences of surgery.

Physical rehabilitation

Physiotherapy. Although the incidence of severe arm and shoulder disorders after mastectomy has largely declined as radical procedures are now seldom performed, minor nerve damage may still occur, and thus physiotherapy should be started as soon as possible after surgery. A range of exercises can be used to improve arm and shoulder mobility (Table 8.1). The patient should be able to brush the back of her hair and fasten zips at the back of her clothing by the time she returns home, and exercises should be continued after discharge from hospital. Physiotherapy can also reduce the risk of lymphedema after full axillary

TABLE 8.1

Exercises to improve arm and shoulder mobility after surgery for breast cancer

Perform each of these exercises three times a day, five to ten times each.

Hair-brushing exercise

Rest your elbow on a table. Keep your head erect. Start by brushing one side only, then gradually increase to your whole head. Be persistent, but don't overdo it.

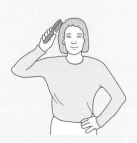

Rope/string exercise

Attach a rope to the door knob or handle. Make small circles with the rope, moving your entire arm from the shoulder, five times in one direction and five times in the other. Gradually increase the size of circle (by moving in closer) and the number of circles.

Arm-swinging exercise

Place your unaffected arm on the back of a chair and rest your forehead on your arm. Allow your other arm to hang loosely and swing it from the shoulder, forwards and backwards, then side to side and in small circles. As the arm relaxes, increase the length of swings and the size of circles. Swing until your arm is relaxed.

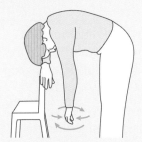

Bra-fastening exercise

Extend your arms, drop your hands from your elbows, then slowly reach behind your back to bra level.

Wall-climbing exercise

Stand with your feet apart for balance. Stand close to and facing a wall. Start with your hands at shoulder level and gradually work them up the wall. Slide your hands back to shoulder level before starting the exercise again. Do this slowly several times a day. Mark the spot reached and aim higher each time.

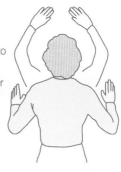

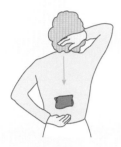

Bean-bag exercise

Drop a bean bag (or a small purse or cosmetic bag) from your right hand over your right shoulder into your left hand at the back. Repeat five times and then change sides.

Rope–pulley exercise

Throw a rope or dressing gown cord over the top of an open door. Sit with the door between your legs. Hold the lower end of the rope in the hand on the side of your surgery and gently pull the other end. Raise your arm as high as possible each time, until it is fully raised.

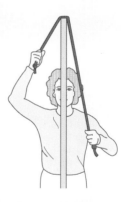

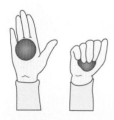

Hand exercise

Alternately squeeze and release a rubber ball or something similar in your hand.

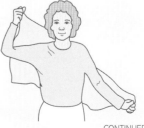

Back-drying exercise

Using a towel, make gentle movements as if drying your back. Repeat on the other side.

CONTINUED

TABLE 8.1 continued

Shoulder-circling exercise

Sit down with your hands in your lap. Circle your shoulders forward or backward, whichever is more comfortable.

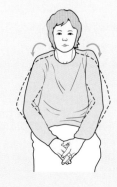

Bent-arm exercise

Sit with your hands on your shoulders. Raise your elbows upwards until you feel a slight pull, and then lower them again. You can support your elbow on the operation side with the other hand if this is more comfortable.

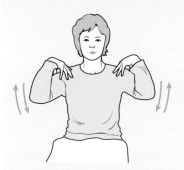

Shoulder-stretching exercise

Hold your hands behind your back. Slowly stretch your arms upwards, and gently lower them again.

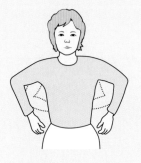

Arm-lift exercise

Lie on the floor with your shoulders relaxed and your hands together in front of you. Raise your arms up over your head, keeping your elbows straight. Gently lower your arms and repeat.

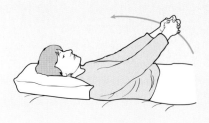

clearance. Elastic bandaging may also be useful, and the affected arm should be elevated whenever possible, particularly at night, and protected from knocks.

Breast prostheses. The use of an appropriate prosthesis is an important aspect of physical rehabilitation after mastectomy, and can also strongly influence psychological rehabilitation. A light, temporary prosthesis can be used for the first few weeks until the wound has healed. A suitable permanent prosthesis can then be selected from the wide range available (Figure 8.1), according to the required size, shape and adherence to the chest wall. Many hospitals have a nurse or physiotherapist trained in the use of breast prostheses.

Psychological rehabilitation. Breast cancer imposes considerable psychological stress and trauma. The initial diagnosis and preparation for surgery can produce a period of emotional turmoil in which rapid mood swings are accompanied by immense disruption to the woman's lifestyle. By contrast, the patient may be euphoric during the immediate postoperative period, possibly due to relief of uncertainty and anticipation of a return to normal life. This initial reaction, however, is transient, and many women experience a period of shock and denial,

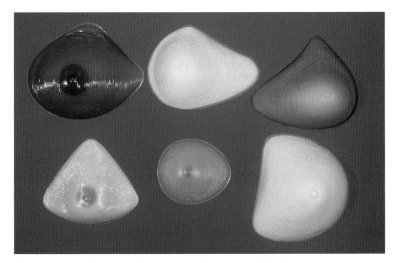

Figure 8.1 A wide range of breast prostheses is available for mastectomy patients.

followed by anxiety, about 2–3 months after surgery. Most women eventually develop coping skills, enabling them to live a normal lifestyle. Approximately 20–30% of women, however, have persistent psychological or sexual problems 1–2 years after surgery, compared with 10% of age-matched women without breast cancer. This does not seem to be related to the type of operation undergone; anxiety and depression appear to be as common in women undergoing conservative surgery as in women undergoing mastectomy.

It is possible that while women undergoing conservative surgery are less concerned about the mutilating effect of surgery and perceived loss of femininity, they are more worried than mastectomy patients about the possibility of recurrence. Patients may also experience anxiety or depression in association with follow-up visits to the clinic, because of the fear that the cancer might recur. If recurrent disease is detected, the patient must again come to terms with the risk of death and the need for further treatment; major depression may occur in up to 50% of women with recurrent disease.

Psychological support is available from a number of sources:

- nurse counselors
- volunteers
- self-help groups
- national organizations.

Specialist nurse counselors can offer advice and emotional support throughout the processes of diagnosis and treatment, and can identify patients with psychological problems requiring treatment. It is important, however, that both the patient and the nurse recognize when such support is no longer needed; maintaining contact on a purely routine basis can foster a sense of being unwell in the patient, making her feel that she is unable to cope on her own. Volunteer groups, composed of women who have had breast cancer themselves, self-help groups and national cancer charities can also offer valuable help and advice to breast cancer patients and their families.

Key points – follow-up and rehabilitation

- Conventional belief in the need for intensive follow-up after completed treatment for primary breast cancer is being challenged by less interventional approaches.
- Attention must be paid to both physical and psychological rehabilitation.
- Simple physical exercises, initiated early, accelerate and improve rehabilitation.
- Emotional and spiritual support should not be overlooked.

Key references

Fallowfield L, Jenkins V. Communication of sad, bad and difficult news. *Lancet* 2004;363: 312–19.

GIVIO Investigators. Impact of follow-up testing on survival and health-related quality of life in breast cancer patients. *JAMA* 1994;271: 1587–92.

Rosselli Del Turco M, Palli D, Cariddi A et al. for the National Research Council Project on Breast Cancer Follow-up. Intensive diagnostic follow-up after treatment of primary breast cancer. *JAMA* 1994;271:1593–7.

The term 'advanced breast cancer' refers to stage III (locally advanced, unsuitable for surgery) and stage IV (metastatic) disease, which are incurable by surgery. Thus, the aims of treatment in advanced breast cancer are palliation – to control symptoms of both primary disease and metastases – and prolongation of life where possible. This means that the treatment strategy should be tailored to the needs of the individual patient. Usually the two aims are compatible, but they may conflict, so sensitivity to the patient's wishes and view of life is paramount.

When cure is only remotely possible, careful, explicit goal-setting becomes of the essence. What is the purpose of treatment, and should it be given now or later? What do symptoms mean, and should they be managed as specific symptoms or as indicators of a required change in the systemic approach? What comorbidities exist? How do they interact with the malignancy? What is the social setting? Management of the disease is not only treatment; it requires balancing of all of these issues.

Perhaps there is one useful rule of thumb. Breast cancer is a chronic and recurrent disease. In an individual patient, the best predictor of the future is the past. Slowly growing disease before diagnosis and a long disease-free interval after primary treatment are hallmarks of a process fundamentally different from the more explosive presentations, such as inflammatory lesions and progression during adjuvant therapy. In general, a remission is one-half as likely as a primary response, and the duration is one-third to one-half the length.

Evaluation of advanced cancer
Patients with advanced breast cancer may show a variety of symptoms (Table 9.1), and thus a careful evaluation is necessary to determine the most appropriate treatment.

Treatment of local symptoms
High-energy radiotherapy is generally used in patients with locally advanced disease to prevent skin ulceration, reduce tumor size and

TABLE 9.1

Symptoms of advanced breast cancer

- Patients with locally advanced disease may show peau d'orange, infiltration of the skin and, occasionally, ulceration. Lymphedema may lead to swelling of the arm; involvement of axillary nerves may result in pain or paralysis of the arm

- Bone metastases may present as bone pain or pathological fractures. Hypercalcemia due to bone metastases results in weakness and lethargy, nausea and vomiting, constipation and general malaise

- Lung metastases may give rise to pleural effusion, leading to breathlessness

- Liver metastases produce nausea, anorexia, weight loss and jaundice

- Metastases in the skull or brain can cause an increase in intracranial pressure, resulting in headaches and neurological symptoms such as fits or disturbances in speech or movement

lessen the involvement of the chest wall. A dose of 40–50 Gy is normally given in 15–25 fractions over 3–5 weeks. The most common side effects are lethargy and skin reactions. Such treatment produces good remission rates, but only about 30% of patients remain free from local disease at death with radiotherapy alone. However, a combination of systemic treatment (see below) and radiotherapy increases the initial response rate to over 80%.

Mastectomy is normally avoided in women with locally advanced breast cancer because local recurrence occurs rapidly and may make palliation more difficult. By contrast, surgery may be useful to prevent skin ulceration in women with metastatic disease and a reasonable life expectancy.

Systemic treatment

Systemic therapy can delay disease progression and improve symptoms in 30–70% of patients. In general, hormones are the best first choice when the prognostic evidence is supportive (postmenopause, long disease-free interval, hormone receptor positive disease, bony disease). Tamoxifen has been the mainstay of treatment in this group of women, though the aromatase inhibitors are coming into wider use. Premenopausal women are most likely to benefit from chemotherapy. There are, however, individual exceptions, as well as an increasing tendency to combine both modes of treatment. Cultural and geographic differences in treatment approach also exist, particularly in the 'grey zones' of scientific knowledge: the North American preference is for cytotoxic chemotherapy, while Europe tends to use hormones.

Endocrine therapy in premenopausal women consists of ovarian ablation, which was traditionally achieved by ovariectomy or radiation treatment of the ovaries. Because of the morbidity associated with these techniques, however, GnRH analogs such as goserelin are increasingly being used. These drugs, given monthly by depot injection, block estrogen secretion by inhibiting the release of luteinizing hormone. Side effects include pain or swelling at the injection site, hot flashes and gastrointestinal disturbances. Tamoxifen is also being increasingly used for palliation in premenopausal women because of its good tolerability.

Second-line therapy may be possible in postmenopausal patients who relapse after treatment with tamoxifen or other agents. With the newer aromatase inhibitors, some of the problems and the often significant side effects of the first compounds have been overcome, including a troublesome rash with an earlier version of aminoglutethimide. In randomized controlled trials, anastrozole produced the same degree of second-line response, but with some advantages in tolerability and possibly a small survival advantage compared with megestrol acetate. On the basis of the data currently available, it seems likely that the aromatase inhibitors will supplant tamoxifen for ER+ve postmenopausal women, particularly in PR–ve and/or *HER2-neu*-positive cases.

Synthetic progestogens, such as megestrol acetate, may be useful in some patients, but are associated with significant and often distressing weight gain.

Combination chemotherapy regimens can provide excellent palliation and occasionally durable intermediate-term responses. The principal challenges are which regimen to use, when to switch and how long to persist. Overall response rates are approximately 40–60%, with a median time to relapse of 6–10 months and survivals of 30 months. The occasional, hugely gratifying, long-term sustained response is one of the enigmas of modern oncology.

Typical regimens include:

- cyclophosphamide, methotrexate and fluorouracil
- doxorubicin and cyclophosphamide
- fluorouracil, doxorubicin and cyclophosphamide
- fluorouracil, epirubicin and cisplatin
- taxanes, alone or in combination.

Such regimens are administered approximately monthly, either continuously until progression, or intermittently to control symptoms. While continuous treatment appears to offer some symptomatic advantage, there is no overall survival advantage.

Treatment can, however, be associated with substantial toxicity and thus may severely impair quality of life in patients in whom a remission is not achieved. The relative benefits and risks of treatment must, therefore, be discussed with the patient before starting therapy.

Newer agents. The range of drugs available is constantly expanding. Some are modifications of existing drugs (epirubicin, for example, is an analog of doxorubicin), while others are novel, such as the taxanes, paclitaxel and docetaxel. The taxanes in particular have been the subject of much discussion, and their use is increasing as a result of the substantial response rates reported in heavily pretreated patients. There is some evidence suggesting a modest survival advantage, but, in our opinion, quality of life ought to be the main outcome determinant. Pending such data, new agents should be used cautiously, particularly outside clinical trials, with careful attention to the setting of clear therapeutic goals and the relative likelihood of benefit and side effects.

Trastuzumab is becoming part of the armamentarium in the treatment of advanced disease, perhaps more rapidly in the USA than elsewhere (in the UK it is licensed for use alone or in combination with paclitaxel only). The response rate in heavily pretreated patients is substantial, and occasional dramatic sustained remissions have been reported. Because of the links between *HER2-neu* overexpression, disease aggressiveness and response to the drug, there is intense interest in the development of strategies that better identify those likely to respond. The drug is expensive, somewhat difficult to handle, and is associated with significant risk of cardiac toxicity. Nonetheless, it offers 'proof of concept' and likely heralds a new focus on molecular pathway targeting.

Fulvestrant is a new ER antagonist approved for the treatment of hormone-receptor-positive, metastatic breast cancer in postmenopausal women with disease progression following antiestrogen therapy. It inhibits binding of estradiol to the ER and eventually induces a reduction of cellular ER levels. In clinical trials involving postmenopausal women with advanced breast cancer that had progressed on tamoxifen therapy, fulvestrant has been shown to be at least as effective as anastrozole for several efficacy endpoints, including an increase in mean duration of response. In clinical studies, fulvestrant had a good tolerability profile.

The novel mode of action of fulvestrant means that it offers the potential for further clinical response following resistance to prior endocrine therapies. The appropriate positioning of fulvestrant within sequential endocrine therapies is currently under consideration.

Bone-marrow transplantation. In the USA, recurrent or high-risk early breast cancers were the most common reasons for bone-marrow transplantation (BMT). Technological advances, such as blood-cell-line colony stimulators and harvesting of peripheral stem cells, reduced the risks associated with the technique and, in a few centers, it was even performed as an outpatient procedure. The surge in interest was driven by anecdotal reports and uncontrolled trials, and by the conviction that dose intensity offered a real solution. Unfortunately the trial data, when finally mature, largely dashed the hope. A few clinical trials are exploring the biology of very intensive therapies further, and by rights BMT should be entertained only in that setting.

New strategies. Half a century of concerted research and experience is leading to a new understanding of breast cancer, and old drugs are being used in new ways. In addition to directly attacking the cancer cell, the local environment and the vascular supply (angiogenesis) are being targeted. Drugs such as cyclophosphamide, methotrexate, aspirin and the COX-2 inhibitors are being combined in continuous low doses and provocative responses are being seen.

Treatment of metastatic disease

Metastatic breast cancer may present in many forms. Some of the consequences of metastatic disease warrant emergency treatment because of the risk of death or permanent disability (Table 9.2).

Bone metastases. Localized bone pain can be resolved by a short course of radiotherapy in about 95% of cases. If analgesia is required, simple analgesics such as aspirin or non-steroidal anti-inflammatory drugs (NSAIDs) should be tried first, followed by more potent agents as necessary. Potent analgesics may produce nausea, and so antiemetic treatment should be given concomitantly. Widespread bone pain can be treated by radioactive strontium or sequential upper and lower hemibody radiotherapy. The treatment of bone metastases is summarized in Table 9.3.

Bisphosphonates, such as pamidronate, are a new class of drug that appears to be helpful in bony disease. They work by suppressing osteoclast activity, thus inhibiting bone resorption, and have been shown to be effective and well tolerated in controlling malignant

TABLE 9.2

Oncological emergencies in breast cancer

Suspicion alone of the following conditions warrants immediate specialist attention:

- Spinal cord compression
- Uncontrolled pain
- Cerebral metastases
- Incipient fracture of femur
- Hypercalcemia

TABLE 9.3

Treatment of bone metastases

Localized bone pain

- External beam radiotherapy
- Analgesics
- Non-steroidal anti-inflammatory drugs

Pathological fractures

- Internal fixation and radiotherapy
- Bone gels

Widespread bone pain

- Radioactive strontium
- Sequential hemibody radiotherapy
- Analgesics
- Non-steroidal anti-inflammatory drugs
- Bisphosphonates

hypercalcemia. More recent studies have shown bisphosphonates to delay bony metastatic progression and decrease the incidence of pathological fracture. It is therefore likely that they will be widely used.

Approximately 50% of patients with metastases in the femur experience pathological fractures, and these should be treated by internal fixation followed by radiotherapy; indeed, prophylactic fixation of the femur may be beneficial in patients at risk of fracture. Pathological fractures of the humerus can be treated simply by immobilization of the arm, followed by a short course of radiotherapy. Pathological fractures of the vertebra require urgent treatment with surgery or radiotherapy to prevent the risk of paralysis or urinary incontinence.

Solitary or critically located metastases can on occasion be excised and replaced with bone gels, most typically in the spine.

Involvement of the bone marrow can result in anemia. Short-term improvements can be obtained by blood transfusion; for long-term treatment, high doses of corticosteroids, endocrine therapy or chemotherapy with vinca alkaloids can be given.

Hypercalcemia resulting from bone metastases should be treated urgently by intravenous fluid infusion and forced diuresis to avoid renal impairment. Recurrence can be prevented with corticosteroids. Bisphosphonates, such as pamidronate, are becoming first-line treatment.

Pleural effusion. Breathlessness resulting from pleural effusion can be relieved by chest drainage. However, reaccumulation of fluid occurs in almost all patients owing to the presence of malignant cells in the pleural cavity, and thus local administration (via the chest drain) of agents such as bleomycin, tetracycline or talc is necessary.

Lymphedema. In most women with lymphedema, pain and loss of mobility in the arm can be controlled by measures such as physiotherapy, elastic compression bandages and pneumatic compression.

Liver metastases can be reduced by radiotherapy or high-dose corticosteroids. There have been reports of successful control of liver metastases by local ablative measures such as cryosurgery, ultrasound, electrocoagulation and the injection of vessel-obliterating species such as radioactive yttrium. While these strategies may be locally effective, liver metastases are frequently multiple and associated with overt disease at other sites.

Neurological complications. Patients with cerebral metastases can be treated with high doses of corticosteroids (e.g. dexamethasone, 12–16 mg/day) to relieve edema, followed by fractionated radiotherapy. Most patients, however, survive for only 3–4 months after treatment.

Palliative care in terminal disease

In the final stages of breast cancer, the palliative aim of treatment becomes paramount. Because the natural history of breast cancer is very variable, this phase may last a few days or several months. The most distressing symptoms of terminal breast cancer include:

- pain
- insomnia
- nausea
- constipation
- dyspnea.

Pain is frequently widespread, and may have several causes. Each site and cause of pain should be identified to allow the most effective analgesic to be given. Strong opiates can be used when the pain does not respond to simple analgesics or weak opiates; fear of addiction is unnecessary and, with appropriate dosage intervals, continuous pain relief can be provided. Laxatives should be given concomitantly to prevent constipation. Insomnia and anxiety can be relieved with benzodiazepines, such as temazepam or diazepam. Dyspnea is an under-reported symptom in terminal disease, for which appropriate interventions are available and appreciated.

The WHO has introduced the concept of the pain ladder (Figure 9.1) in the management of cancer pain. This concept involves the use of a variety of agents, ranging from simple analgesics to opiates, depending on the site and severity of pain.

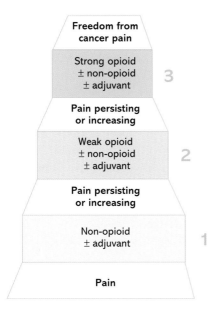

Figure 9.1

The pain ladder.

> **Key points – management of advanced cancer**
>
> - Site of recurrence, extent, time to recurrence and evaluation of comorbidities are critical determinants of prognosis and treatment.
> - Explicit goal-setting for patients and health professionals is essential.
> - Oncological emergencies must be anticipated and recognized.
> - Effective pain management is almost always possible.

Spiritual and emotional support

At best, modern medical treatment can postpone death from advanced breast cancer to a limited extent, but there is a tendency to overmedicalize the terminal stages of the disease. In addition to symptomatic treatment, it is also important to remember the patient's emotional needs. Sooner or later we all have to recognize that, just as there is a time to be born, so there is a time to die. One of the greatest tragedies we can witness is the desperate patient, supported by her desperate relatives, seeking out magic cures at great expense in futile attempts to delay the inevitable.

It is essential that health professionals recognize the need for spiritual and emotional support for the dying patient. While all doctors should, of course, be taught the skills of listening and counseling, no breast cancer team is complete without access to a professionally trained counselor or the appropriate ministers of religion. Coming to terms with the inevitability of death may have a calming influence and may even reduce the need for pharmacological support. The hospice movement pioneered in the UK is an example of this ethos at work and has now been copied in many countries around the world.

Key references

Chang, JC, Wooten, EC, Tsimelzon A et al. Gene expression profiling for the prediction of therapeutic response to docetaxel in patients with breast cancer. *Lancet* 2003;362:362–9.

Cherny NI, Portenoy RK. Cancer pain management. *Cancer* 1993; 72:3393–415.

Coates A, Gebski V, Bishop JF et al. Improving the quality of life during chemotherapy for advanced breast cancer. A comparison of intermittent and continuous treatment strategies. *N Engl J Med* 1987;317:1490–5.

Levy MH. Pharmacologic treatment of cancer pain. *N Engl J Med* 1996; 335:1124–32.

Wong K, Henderson IC. Management of metastatic breast cancer. *World J Surg* 1994; 18:98–111.

The clinical trial process may be our most powerful analytical tool for developing new treatments, and is increasingly used, especially in oncology. There is also good evidence that the trial process itself raises the quality of care. However, a good trial must ask a good question and be structured to provide a reasonable chance of getting a good answer. Bad questions and poor execution defeat the purpose. It must also be remembered that no trial can supplant good clinical observation.

Should my patient enter a trial?

Many patients attending specialist centers are recruited into trials, and they often turn to their family physician for advice. Should they enter a trial? – By all means, if the question is good, the design makes an answer feasible, and entry does not compromise the individual patient's care. However, clinical trials place a burden on all involved, because the data must be meticulously collected and analyzed; a good trial design will make this as easy as possible.

Trials can also be frustrating because the 'answer' will not be known until the study is complete. If your patient is one of the first to be entered into a trial with a 5-year follow-up, then – barring an unexpectedly dramatic result – you may not know the outcome for a decade.

Finally, an admission of uncertainty by the physician is implicit in a randomized trial, which can be difficult for some patients (and physicians) to accept.

Characteristics of clinical trials

The purpose of a clinical trial is to conduct a human experiment that is likely to provide an answer to a clinical or a biological question (or both). Although there are regional differences in the extent of informed consent required and its documentation, three fundamental principles apply.

- The trial must address a legitimate question to which the answer is currently unclear. In a randomized trial, this introduces the concept of 'equipoise', which means that each arm of the study has equal merit in advance of the experiment.

- The patient must be an informed and willing participant in the study.
- The patient may decline to enter the trial, or withdraw at any time during the study, without prejudicing their subsequent care.

There are four clinical trial structures, each of which has a different purpose.

The Phase I study provides basic pharmacological and toxicological information. It is not a test of therapeutic efficacy. For drugs with relatively non-toxic mechanisms of action (e.g. endocrine agents), Phase I studies may be carried out in healthy volunteers; trials on cancer chemotherapy agents are almost always conducted in major cancer centers with patients whose illness is progressive despite all available treatment. Phase I studies are usually not randomized.

The Phase II study uses Phase I data to select a range of doses. The sample size is usually 15–20 patients, but may be increased if a major response is observed. The patients usually have end-stage disease, and may have previously received many other drugs. A Phase II study may test drug combinations. It is usually not randomized.

The Phase III study is a randomized trial comparing the effects of different treatments, one of which represents the current 'state of the art'. Typical outcome measures are survival, disease-free survival, response, toxicity and quality of life. Because the differences in outcome between groups are often expected to be small, these trials involve many patients; they are conducted over several years and involve many institutions in many different countries.

The Phase IV study is less commonly encountered. Its aim is to evaluate the long-term consequences of an established treatment. In the pharmaceutical industry, such a trial might be referred to as a postmarketing study.

Manufacturers' trials. The purpose may be to achieve regulatory approval, or advance the market position of the drug or device in question. Such trials are subject to the same ethical guidelines and constraints as others. In the fractious world of clinical research there is a tendency to 'take sides' with or against the drug industry. Both good and poor trials can be mounted by either group.

Clinical research groups' trials. Within the last 3 years the UK Department of Health has established a National Cancer Research Network (NCRN) to encourage clinical trial activity. One of its stated aims is to raise recruitment from 3% to 10% of eligible cancer patients; indirectly, this endorses the process as integral to good clinical practice. The NCRN can already boast a 7% accrual rate. This mirrors numerous national and regional efforts to accrue patients rapidly and advance clinical science. In the USA there are several large clinical trials groups, including the Southwestern Oncology Group (SWOG), the National Surgical Adjuvant Breast and Bowel Program (NSABP), and the Eastern Co-operative Oncology Group (ECOG), to name a few. In Canada, the Canadian National Cancer Institute (NCI(C)) is the leading agency. There are similar groups in Australia and in mainland Europe.

In recent years even these large organizations have begun to pool efforts globally, both to increase the accrual rate and to advance the generalizability of the result. These clinical research groups are academically based, and closely linked to governmental research agencies. The compounds and strategies being tested come from laboratory research involving both public and private sectors. Generally the investigational agents are provided by the government or the pharmaceutical company without cost to the patient or institution.

Stopping rules

Patient safety is of primary concern in a trial. It is possible that a new treatment may harbor an unanticipated disadvantage or that treatments compared may have much greater differences in effect than anticipated. Such concerns are addressed by interim analysis of blinded data, with rules to shut down a trial and make the results public if either of these events occur. These are not easy systems to design or execute. There is great pressure from all directions to get the data early. The risk is losing important long-term information. This issue is particularly important in the adjuvant setting, where much breast cancer research and treatment is concentrated. The controversy reached a public boiling point when a *Sunday New York Times* editorial called the early closing of an adjuvant aromatase inhibitor trial 'ethical overkill'. The trial designer must therefore give very careful thought to all the outcome considerations in a trial and to the early estimators which are used. It is our view that the referring physician, consultant and patient must understand these stopping rules, at least in outline.

Future of the trials process

The Human Genome Project and the study of derived proteins (proteomics) raise the prospect of ever more precisely engineered drugs. In the USA, a fast-track mechanism for cancer and other 'emergency' diseases has accelerated the introduction of new drugs. The trials process will thus gain even greater importance in the advance of medicine.

There will be consequences for every clinician's practice. For example, genetic prediction (e.g. *BRCA1/2*) will lead to proposed interventions before the disease even becomes apparent, and possibly before the early transforming event. These trials will involve large numbers of 'worried well', and will require long follow-up and expanded scrutiny for unintended adverse effects. Another consequence is that target groups will be smaller, so trials will become less centralized, raising questions about quality control and adequate surveillance.

There is a vague but troublesome generic risk: the new model is based on a new paradigm and neither is fully validated. That carries with it the risk of systematic error in trial design, conduct and interpretation. This happened in the 1970s, as exemplified by the thalidomide episode, and to a lesser extent more recently with gene therapies. For the period of instability which is likely to come, vigilance about design, conduct and oversight will be especially necessary.

Key points – clinical trials

- The well-conducted clinical trial remains the benchmark of both therapy and medical progress.
- You should ask questions and conduct personal due diligence about trials in which your patients' participation is proposed.

Key references

Early Breast Cancer Trialists' Collaborative Group. Effects of adjuvant tamoxifen and of cytotoxic therapy on mortality in early breast cancer. An overview of 61 randomized trials among 28 896 women. *N Engl J Med* 1988;319:1681–92.

Early Breast Cancer Trialists' Collaborative Group. Systemic treatment of early breast cancer by hormonal, cytotoxic or immune therapy. 133 randomised trials involving 31 000 recurrences and 24 000 deaths among 75 000 women (Part I). *Lancet* 1992;339:1–15.

Early Breast Cancer Trialists' Collaborative Group. Tamoxifen for early breast cancer: an overview of the randomised trials. *Lancet* 1998;351:1451–67.

Howell A, Dowsett M. Recent advances in endocrine therapy of breast cancer. *BMJ* 1997;315:863–6.

Kmietowicz Z. Deaths from breast cancer fall dramatically in UK and US. *BMJ* 2000;320:1428.

Peto R, Pike MC, Armitage P. Design and analysis or randomized clinical trials requiring prolonged observation of each patient. I. Introduction and design. *Br J Cancer* 1976;34:585–612.

Slutsky AS, Lavery JV. Data safety and monitoring boards. *N Engl J Med* 2004;350:1143–7.

Reconceptualization

One hundred and fifty years ago, microscopy and tissue staining revealed that cancers started in a tissue of origin, invaded and metastasized. At the same time, Koch and his generation observed microbes, establishing the idea of the foreign invader as the cause of illness, and thence the dominant therapeutic strategy of eliminating the invader by killing it. This concept was also adopted in the treatment of cancer: the malignant mass was seen as curable only by eliminating the last cell. The Halsted principle of centrifugal progression of a localized breast neoplasm was elucidated in 1907 and spawned half a century of ever more extensive surgery, limited only by technology.

However, over the last 20 years, evidence that contradicts this paradigm has accumulated (Boxes 11.1–11.3). Those treating advanced breast cancer with hormones seemed to see responses qualitatively similar to those achieved with the newer chemotherapies, yet hormones were not known as cytotoxic agents. Small doses of 5-fluorouracil and methotrexate were found to produce a persistent disease-free and

---

Box 11.1

One would expect a constant hazard rate for the appearance of distant metastases from the point of initial diagnosis and treatment. However, clinical experience reveals a peak hazard for recurrence at about three years after diagnosis and treatment, with the suggestion of a second peak at seven to nine years after treatment. Furthermore, in disease that is more advanced at presentation, we do not observe an earlier peak but merely a greater amplitude of peak hazard in the same period. Finally, the most extreme example for peak hazard rates is seen among young women with breast cancer: it appears that, if they survive the first three or four years, then their risk of relapse and death is extremely low.

overall survival advantage. The surgeon Fisher, amongst others, investigated the data like these that did not fit the prevailing paradigm, and theorized that breast cancer is a systemic disease, and the histopathological and nodal characteristics seen at surgery are hallmarks of a process. In other words, unlike Halsted, he viewed surgery as a diagnostic rather than therapeutic technique. At the same time, Sporn began to consider cancer a dynamic process of subtle interaction between what had been considered autonomous tumor cells and the local environment, including the supporting stroma. Fidler elaborated the dynamic and progressive nature of tumor heterogeneity, and Liotta offered experimental evidence, at least in tissue culture, that the process could be up- and downregulated.

A reconceptualization of cancer is now occurring: the idea of a relentlessly progressing, malignant *entity*, largely fixed in its properties, is being challenged by that of a complex, dynamic, ever-changing *equilibrium* of altered growth and metabolism. We suspect that the process we call cancer is a subtle, time-variable, non-linear regulatory process, and is probably field-dependent; in other words, a given molecule may upregulate in one setting, and downregulate in another. The implications of this conceptual change will be profound: if cancer is a potentially remediable disorder of regulation, its ultimate control cannot be achieved by killing all malignant cells, so the strategies used to devise new treatments, and the means of their evaluation, will also change. New drugs will achieve their effects not by killing cells, but by reregulating them. Defective communication pathways will have to be reset or bypassed. Microenvironments that stimulate proliferation will have to be retuned.

We believe that most organs in the body produce latent cancers whose prevalence increases with age. These latent lesions, resulting from an accumulation of molecular events linked to a temporary failure of DNA repair, are a necessary but not sufficient condition for invasive cancer. They are sufficiently common in the breast, prostate and thyroid to suggest that all adults harbor cancer at some time. We think that, if left undetected, these cancers will exist in dynamic equilibrium with surrounding tissue for years until stochastic events, either adverse or favorable, lead to their progression to an invasive phenotype or return to normal. Adverse events might include further molecular damage, direct or indirect trauma leading to the activation of wound repair genes and angiogenesis, or even minor systemic disturbance such as may result from psychological trauma (see Box 11.2). Central to our understanding of this process is the recent work on pro- and antiangiogenic cytokines, pro- and antiproliferation cytokines and pro- and antiapoptopic signaling proteins. These provide a 'soup' within which a latent primary or metastatic focus can remain in a state of dynamic equilibrium, be triggered into progression or even regress to the norm (see Figure 3.2).

Science is a search for understanding, rather than received wisdom. Professional acceptance of new ideas and changes in treatment cannot happen without dogged groundwork and consensus-building. Our understanding of breast cancer is a continuing odyssey. The description and categorization of fixed images and static parameters was an essential step, one that made possible the

---

Box 11.2

The natural history of breast cancer in individual patients is highly capricious. For example:

- A 52-year-old clergyman's wife had a stage 1 breast cancer. The disease recurred after 10 years, just after she entered an affair with a parishioner; it went into remission when the affair ended and she reconciled with her husband, and recurred rapidly and fatally with another liaison. Similar stories relating to psychological and physical trauma are reliably reported from time to time.

- On mammographic screening of a 53-year-old nurse, a small focus of microcalcification was detected. The nurse proceeded to stereotactic core-cut biopsy, which revealed intermediate-grade ductal carcinoma in situ; she was advised to have further surgery. She refused for reasons that are not clear, but returned to the clinic 9 months later with a breast full of invasive carcinoma. This case is far removed from our usual experiences of the natural history of ductal carcinoma in situ.

next step, in which we are coming to understand cancer as a dynamic process.

Prevention

On current evidence, we know that genetic predisposition plays a role in breast cancer. For some, such as those harboring *BRCA1* or *BRCA2*, it is pervasive. For most it is a small multiplier of relative risk.

Current preventive approaches reflect the anatomic consequences of the disease rather than genetic understanding (hence prophylactic mastectomy and oophorectomy). However, as the functional consequences of the genetics become clear, so will strategies to redress the mutation, such as drugs and advice on changing lifestyle to avoid enhancing behaviors.

Several population-based preventive strategies are emerging. Epidemiological evidence that delayed menarche, less body fat in adolescence and fewer ovulatory cycles over a lifetime lead to a reduced risk of female reproductive tract cancers has resulted in recommendations to increase youth fitness and exercise levels. As a considerably more interventionist step, there is also work towards modification of the oral contraceptive.

However, the tendency to intervene early in the cancer induction process will have to be tempered by the realization that, for every breast cancer that is prevented or delayed, many women will undertake treatment whose effects may not become apparent for a generation. Advanced disease may represent an end stage of the failure of control mechanisms in early disease, and thus be a very poor model for innovative therapy. In the short term, our zeal to identify risk factors must be tempered with the realization that therapies extrapolated from advanced disease settings may have only limited value.

Early diagnosis

There is still much controversy over early diagnosis and screening (see Box 11.3). Even in postmenopausal women the benefit is not as great as hoped. In absolute terms we have to screen 1250 women for 10 years to save one life. Against that there are undoubted cases

> **Box 11.3**
>
> Screening for breast cancer remains extremely controversial. Put simply, the benefits are less than predicted by the biological models on which screening rests: progressive tumor growth and an irreversibly deranged genome. If the theory were translated into clinical fact, then we would expect that with the increasing detection of ductal carcinoma in situ in all age groups, there would be a decline in the subsequent incidence of invasive breast cancer and along with this a substantial reduction in breast cancer mortality. This is simply not the case. The introduction of screening has led worldwide to an increased recorded incidence of the disease, with 20% of the cases detected being in situ, and yet with little or no detectable decline in the rates of invasive disease. Furthermore, the benefits for postmenopausal women are modest, with estimates in the range of 18–25% relative risk reduction, whereas for premenopausal women the most recent meta-analysis has shown an excess of breast cancer deaths in the first three years after entry into the screening programme.

where cancers are detected 'too early', that is, low-grade DCIS, which if left undisturbed might spontaneously regress, or if biopsied might progress owing to the induction of angiogenesis as a wounding response. Complicating matters further, we now begin to appreciate that early cancers are different from later ones.

The anatomic approach to early diagnosis will eventually be superseded by tests that detect abnormal function. Genetic testing for susceptibility, positron emission tomography (PET) and PET-MRI linking anatomy to function are early examples. Proteomics, the emerging study of the proteins produced by genes, may offer another approach.

Treatment

Several principles have been established in the treatment of evident disease, but their application is still to be optimized.

- Given good technique, lesser surgery with radiation provides better cosmesis, and a recurrence and survival outcome equivalent to breast removal. Many women still opt for mastectomy, some due to the inconvenience imposed by radiation treatments. Newer approaches to radiation may relieve that concern.
- Broader use of sentinel node sampling provides adequate prognostic information without the consequences of full axillary dissection. As we shift from anatomic to functional staging, this requirement may also be relieved.
- Systemic treatment for breast cancer is now fully established. An expanded range of agents is available for hormone-sensitive breast cancers. Timing, duration and sequence will continue to be debated.
- For premenopausal women and cancers that are not hormone-sensitive, systemic cytotoxics remain the mainstay. Addition of the anthracyclines and taxanes to the established CMF regimen has increased the proportionate disease-free response rates by 10–15%. The trend is to extend the length of treatment, the enthusiasm for highly intensive therapies having been dampened by experience. Large trials will be required because the anticipated differences will be small.

A new range of options is now becoming available from the areas of molecular and genetic medicine.

- Therapies aimed at altering the host side of the tumor–host symbiosis will reach the clinic, for example antiangiogenesis strategies.
- Small molecules are being developed, narrowly targeted to proliferation enzymes, such as matrix metalloproteinases, which have a role in invasion. Some 600 such compounds are in development. Like trastuzumab, these drugs will be employed on a functional basis. Tests for overexpression of the target pathway will be linked to drug use and monitoring.

Without doubt, the defining challenge will be when to treat and for how long. Do we intervene at the first expression of a precursor process or wait until a mass is present? It depends on the mode of action and efficacy of our treatment. The answers to the question require a fuller framing of the regulatory model. One scenario would have a series of interventions very early on for those at highest risk – a next-generation application of the tamoxifen and raloxifene chemoprevention trials. Later intervention would be the strategy for small lesions that may be reversible with antiangiogenic agents, for example. Contemporary ablative approaches like cytotoxics and radiation would be used for larger tumors.

Key references

Fidler IJ, Hart IR. Biological diversity in metastatic neoplasms: Origins and implications. *Science* 1982:217: 998–1003.

Fisher B. The evolution of paradigms for the management of breast cancer: A personal perspective. *Cancer Res* 1992;52:2371–83.

Liotta LA, Steeg PS, Stetler-Stevenson WG. Cancer metastasis and angiogenesis: An imbalance of positive and negative regulation. *Cell* 1991;64:327–36.

Schipper H, Baum M, Turley EA. A new biological framework for cancer research. *Lancet* 1996;348: 1149–51.

Schipper H, Goh CR, Wang TL: Rethinking cancer: Should we control rather than kill? Part 1. *Can J Oncol* 1993;3:207–16.

Schipper H, Goh CR, Wang TL. Rethinking cancer: Should we control rather than kill? Part 2. *Can J Oncol* 1993;3:220–24.

Sporn MB. Carcinogenesis and cancer: Different perspectives on the same disease. *Cancer Res* 1991;51: 6215–18.

Useful addresses

Adjuvant!

www.adjuvantonline.com
This site, designed for professionals and extensively updated in early 2004, aggregates data from many trials, particularly the Oxford Overviews, and provides patient-specific estimators of the impact of systemic interventions.

The Canadian Breast Cancer Network

www.cbcn.ca
Treatment guidelines and information for both patients and professionals.

CancerBACUP (UK)

3 Bath Place, Rivington Street
London EC2A 3JR
Helpline (UK only): 0808 800 1234
Tel: +44 (0)20 7696 9003
Fax: +44 (0)20 7696 9002
www.cancerbacup.org.uk
Information for both patients and professionals; helpline includes interpreting service for 12 languages.

CancerNet (USA)

National Cancer Institute
Department of Health and
Human Services
United States Government
www.nci.nih.gov
Possibly the most comprehensive site of all, from a US perspective.

Cancer Research UK

PO Box 123, Lincoln's Inn Fields
London WC2A 3PX
Tel: +44 (0)20 7242 0200
Fax: +44 (0)20 7269 3100
www.cancerresearchuk.org

Frenchay Breast Care Centre (UK)

www.frenchaybreast.co.uk

Minervation (UK)

www.minervation.com/cancer/breast/
professional/
National Electronic Library for Health information on breast cancer.

National Breast Cancer Centre (Australia)

www.nbcc.org.au

The National Breast Cancer Coalition (USA)

1101 17th Street NW, Suite 1300
Washington DC 20036 USA
Tel: 800 622 2838
Tel: +1 202 296 7477
Fax: +1 202 265 6854
www.stopbreastcancer.org

Wellspring (Canada)

www.wellspring.ca
An excellent source of patient and family information.

Index

What the reviewers say:

concise and well written and accompanied by numerous excellent color illustrations... an excellent little book! Score: 100 - 5 Stars

On *Fast Facts – Sexual Dysfunct*
in *Doody's Health Sciences Review*, 2(

it really demystifies the treatments behind this psychiatric disorder

On *Fast Facts – Bipolar Disorders*
in *Doody's Health Sciences Review*, 2004

a timely and accessible book...
a worthwhile and handy tool for medical students

On *Fast Facts – Dyspepsia*, in *Digestive and Liver Disease* 36, 2004

provides a lot of information in a concise and easily accessible format...
a practical guide to managing most lower respiratory tract infections

On *Fast Facts – Respiratory Tract Infection*,
in *Respiratory Care* 49(1), 2004

an invaluable guide to the latest thinking

On *Fast Facts – Irritable Bowel Syndrome*, in *Update*, 4 September 2003

a rapid guide to understanding dementia...
value for money and I would definitely recommend it

On *Fast Facts – Dementia*, in *South African Medical Journal* 93(10), 2003

excellent coverage of symptoms and diagnosis

On *Fast Facts – Dyspepsia*, in *Update*, 19 June, 2003

will likely be read cover to cover in just one or
two sittings by all who are fortunate enough
to obtain a copy

On *Fast Facts – Benign Prostatic Hyperplasia*, 4th edn, in *Doody's Health Sciences Review*, Dec 2002

explains the important facts and demonstrates
the levels of "good practice" that can be achieved

On *Fast Facts – Minor Surgery*,
in *Journal of the Royal Society for the Promotion of Health* 122(3), 2002

a splendid publication

On *Fast Facts – Sexually Transmitted Infections*, in *Journal of Antimicrobial Chemotherapy* 49, 2002

I would highly recommend it
without reservation… 5 stars!

On *Fast Facts – Psychiatry Highlights 2001–02*,
in *Doody's Health Sciences Review*, Sept 2002

I enthusiastically recommend this
stimulating, short book which should
be required reading for all clinicians

On *Fast Facts – Irritable Bowel Syndrome*, in *Gastroenterology* 120(6), 2001

***** outstanding

On *Fast Facts – HIV in Obstetrics and Gynecology*, in *Journal of Pelvic Surgery*, 2001

a gem for family physicians because of its ease
of use and the sophisticated, concise treatment

On *Fast Facts – Epilepsy*, in *American Family Physician* 64(5), 2001

www.fastfacts.com